MORAINE VALLEY COMMUNITY COLLEGE LIBRARY
PALOS HILLS, ILLINOIS

P9-APE-293

MORAINE VALLEY COMMUNITY COLLEGE

3 5029 00402198 4

[WITHDRAWN

RC 553 .A88 T435 2013

Teaching social skills to
people with autism

Teaching Social Skills to People with Autism

Teaching Social Skills to People with Autism

Best Practices in Individualizing Interventions

Edited by Andy Bondy, Ph.D. & Mary Jane Weiss, Ph.D., BCBA-D

Woodbine House **2013**

© 2013 Andy Bondy and Mary Jane Weiss

Cover photo by Steve Liss.

First edition

All rights reserved. Published in the United States of America by Woodbine House, Inc., 6510 Bells Mill Road, Bethesda, MD 20817. 800-843-7323. www.woodbinehouse.com

Library of Congress Cataloging-in-Publication Data

Teaching social skills to people with autism : best practices in individualizing interventions / edited by Andy Bondy, Ph.D., & Mary Jane Weiss, Ph.D., BCBA-D. -- First edition.
    pages cm
 Includes bibliographical references and index.
 ISBN 978-1-60613-011-7
 1. Autistic people--Rehabilitation. 2. Autistic people--Life skills guides. 3. Social skills--Therapeutic use. I. Bondy, Andy, editor of compilation. II. Weiss, Mary Jane, editor of compilation.
  RC553.A88.T435 2013
  616.85'88206--dc23

                                        2013022745

Manufactured in the United States of America

10   9   8   7   6   5   4   3   2   1

Table of Contents

Acknowledgments

Andy thanks Lori, children, and grandchildren for their support—and for their ongoing efforts to improve his social skills!

Mary Jane thanks her friends and family—especially BB, Liam, Nora, and Julia— for their patience, love, and laughter.

Mary Jane and Andy thank everyone at Woodbine House for their assistance at every stage of this book, and especially Susan Stokes, for her expert editing. They also both thank each of the contributors for their patience throughout this project, for their inspiring chapters, and for their dedication to helping all of us teach social skills in more efficient and effective ways.

Introduction

Impairments in social skills (including play skills) remain one of the hallmark features associated with individuals with autism spectrum disorder (ASD). This book is designed to provide readers with advice from experts in the field of ASD, all of whom have extensive backgrounds and histories in developing and evaluating treatment approaches aimed at improved social skills with this population. We asked each author to address the same key issues within each chapter, thus giving an overall structure to each chapter. Some of the areas covered include:

- What is a "social skill?" How are these skills distinguished from language/communication skills?
- What are the key issues associated with assessment and measurement of such skills?
- What are the most effective teaching strategies and how can you train staff and parents to implement these strategies?
- How do you collect and analyze data associated with strategies and progress?
- How do you promote generalization of specific skills?

We believe that the chapter authors provide an excellent array of guidelines involving a host of important skills. Each chapter provides descriptions of essential teaching strategies and the evidence-basis for the authors' suggested strategies. Each chapter also provides several case examples showing how these strategies can be applied to individuals with ASD.

In a very well written and organized chapter, Bridget A. Taylor, from the Alpine Learning Group, opens with a clear discussion about what social skills are and why they are so important in life. She also describes the situations under which particular behaviors are deemed social, as well as the situations under which the mere absence of them is problematic. Taylor then spells out clear guidelines for assessment and goal selection for people with ASD. She also offers a rich array of strategies to effectively teach social skills, including those associated with motivational variables. Taylor provides an excellent review of the evidence basis for a host of strategies. Her chapter ends with a review of several critical issues, including generalization, data collection and analysis, and social validity.

Shahla Ala'i-Rosales, Samantha Cermak, and Kristín Guðmundsdóttir provide an excellent description of a parent-training program, *Sunny Starts*, which was developed at the Department of Behavior Analysis at the University of North Texas. They begin with an emphasis on a contextual understanding of social skills. A contextual analysis of the social development of children notes the importance of interacting with parents—hence, the accent upon parent training. The acronym DANCE is used to suggest the metaphor of the "social dance" that occurs between parents and their children. Social attending and play are the first key skills addressed by parents in the program. The chapter continues with a description of many other key skills and the sequences in which they are taught.

The next chapter, by Marjorie H. Charlop and Melaura Andree Erickson of the Claremont Autism Center, begins with a review of the social skill impairment faced by many with ASD and a discussion of how these issues change as a function of the child's age and setting. The authors describe the important components of their Center's focus and strategies and their efforts to assure the evidence-basis for each teaching tactic. They address how to select target skills and measure progress on those skills and also describe a number of naturalistic teaching strategies, including video modeling and self-management. They provide several case studies to illustrate how a combination of approaches can be successfully used.

Rebecca MacDonald, from the New England Center for Children (NECC), provides a detailed account of teaching pretend play to children with ASD. After an overview of social referencing and joint attention, she explains why play is a crucial skill to teach and how we can address pretend play as well. MacDonald then provides an excellent review of a series of behaviorally based approaches to teaching, including video modeling. Next, she provides details regarding a specific play curriculum developed at NECC. She also provides explicit examples of promoting generalization of play skills.

Saara Mahjouri and Connie Kasari from the Center for Autism Research and Treatment at UCLA offer strong guidelines aimed at facilitating the social inclusion of children with ASD. They provide information regarding the assessment of early intervention targets as well as the ongoing development of social skills, including the Structured Play Assessment. They then review evidence-based strategies to promote peer engagement. Finally, they describe strategies appropriate to school settings and address social skills that are important throughout the course of life.

The next chapter is by Daniel Openden from the Southwest Autism Research and Resource Center at the Arizona State University. He opens with a frank discussion of social competence and the broad approaches of Pivotal Response Treatment and Natural Language Paradigm. He includes a detailed account of the major pivotal areas related to this approach. He also explains how to address special skill targets and collateral changes associated with untargeted social skills.

Jed Baker, from the Social Skills Training Project, writes about key components related to social skill training. He begins with a review of definitions and measurement issues. Next, Baker distinguishes between applied behavior analysis, cognitive-behavioral approaches, and relationship-based approaches, and discusses the evidence associated with each approach. Finally, he provides a set of guidelines regarding how to use key components from the broad array reviewed to design an effective package for individuals with ASD.

Mary Jane Weiss, coeditor of this book, closes with a chapter reviewing both the current best practices and the many challenges that remain for those concerned with teaching social skills to individuals with ASD. She provides a review of many popular social skill teaching strategies but reminds readers that many of these strategies do not have the level of empirical support assumed by many practitioners. Weiss provides clear examples of what evidence-based truly means and explains which strategies have the best empirical support. The chapter ends with a series of questions that all readers should remember as they read reports and studies dealing with the ever-emerging field of social skill training.

While discussions and recommendations about social skills have abounded since the initial identification of autism spectrum disorders, research on evidence-based practices has lagged significantly behind. Furthermore, our clinical impact on social skills has been modest (compared to other curricular areas). Some strategies have become popular because they "feel right" or have "common-sense" appeal. Fortunately, the contributors to this book are well aware of the scientific responsibility they have regarding suggestions and advice that are offered. Each chapter therefore reviews research in detail, often including limitations associated with particular strategies. In addition to familiarizing yourself with the specific information this book provides regarding assessment and intervention, we urge you to learn the best questions to ask so that as new strategies are developed, you will be able to discern the difference between hype and evidence.

We wish each of you a good and successful journey along the path of improving the social skills of those with an autism spectrum disorder.

Andy Bondy and Mary Jane Weiss

1

Improving the Social Behavior of Children with Autism

Bridget A. Taylor

> *Social behavior arises because one organism is important*
> *to another as part of the environment.*
> —B.F. Skinner (1953, p. 298)

Defining "Social Skills"

Think of the "most social" person you know. What does that person do to give you that impression? Perhaps she's good at conversation, makes friends easily, or is gregarious at parties. Or perhaps he is a good listener, asks insightful questions, or can readily identify another's distress and provide just the right support. Social behavior is complex, and involves the dynamic interaction of a variety of discriminative stimuli and consequences. We know it when we see it, and we can sense its absence—yet a concrete definition of a "social skill" remains elusive. And while experts agree that "social skills" can, and often must, be taught, there is little consensus on just what constitutes social behavior (Romanczyk, White, & Gillis, 2005).

Broadly, a social skill could be considered any response that impacts, in a positive way, interpersonal relations with another person. For example, if, knowing that a friend is ill, you ask how she is feeling, your comment may provide your friend with much-needed comfort, and thereby positively affect the interpersonal relationship you share. But other social skills may have little direct effect on interpersonal relationships. For example, while speaking quietly in the library is a learned social skill that positively affects the wellbeing of others—patrons may then enjoy their books in peace and quiet—it has little to do with interacting in an interpersonal way with another person. At the same time, however, we all recognize such skills as part of a social and cultural fabric we share and observe.

One could likewise posit that a social skill is a response maintained by positive social—rather than tangible—reinforcers: a reciprocal compliment, for example, or an enjoyable interaction with a friend. Nevertheless, some social responses are also maintained by tangible reinforcers. Thus, a child may ask for a cookie by saying, "I want cookie," but his parent may prefer a more socially acceptable request, such as, "May I have a cookie, please?" When a child consistently gets the cookie by using the latter request, he learns that the polite response (a social skill) is more likely to win him the desired cookie. The cookie, in turn, maintains the more socially appropriate response.

To further complicate any effort to define what is "social," some undeniably social responses can be maintained by negative reinforcers. Imagine a college freshman who calls home two times a week to ward off a mid-week call from her mother, who will predictably complain about how infrequently her daughter phones home. Here, the young woman's social initiation is partially maintained by the consequence of avoiding her mother's nagging. Moreover, social skills involve not only readily apparent vocal verbal behavior (e.g., initiating a greeting with an old friend at a party after not seeing him for a long time), but also involve subtle—or not so subtle—nonvocal behaviors, such as standing at the appropriate distance from the person you are talking to, or knowing just how long to look into a person's eyes when you are speaking or listening. And, further still, social skills not only involve *initiating* responses with others, but also the ability to *respond* to others' initiations, and interpret the subtle and unwritten rules of social engagement and provide an appropriate social response. For example, recognizing that your companion is no longer interested in a chosen topic of conversation, or realizing that you have inadvertently insulted someone, are critical social skills, as are the responses that follow.

And while it may make intuitive sense to assume that communication and language skills must be "social skills," that equation does not always hold true. There can be no doubt that communication and social skills overlap, and often significantly. The polite request for a cookie delivers a message, as does the telephone call to an ailing friend. Both responses are communicative and social, even though they lead to different reinforcers. At the same time, however, some language skills may have no direct social value at all. Rehearsing a list of grocery items while on your way to the store is not necessarily social: No one hears your recitation of the list, nor does another act or react on the basis of your utterances. Still, the noncommunicative recitation of the list may play a role in some larger social initiative; perhaps you are shopping for a dinner party, or trying to remember items your ailing friend asked you to pick up at the store.

In addition, some social skills only communicate a message if the social skill is *not* demonstrated. As explained above, it is certainly a social skill to stand an appropriate distance from a conversation partner. That skill, however, has little palpable communicative content—until the norm is violated. Standing too close to another person may indicate aggression, attraction, or rudeness; standing too far away may suggest shyness, or intimidation, or disinterest. Selecting the appropriate conversational distance seems merely neutral. The same is true of lowering one's voice in a library. Adherence to the social norm sends little or no message, while its violation speaks volumes— here, literally. In the end, the interaction of language, communication, and social skills in a given context may not be immediately apparent.

Of course, modern technology continues to shift and transform the boundaries of social behavior. Social skills now include the complex rules of negotiating web-regulated social worlds—to "friend," or not to "friend"?— and the intricacies of differentiating between textual responses appropriate to one medium, yet patently improper to another. Consider the evolving language of text-messaging, in which configurations of standard punctuation marks—say, >:(or ;-p—communicate complex emotional messages by approximating facial expressions. Likewise, the social and communication skills that may generate an avid following on Twitter are worlds away from those of the political blogger. As technology continues to expand, social skills and social repertoires will expand and morph in response, often eluding concretized notions of appropriate social behavior.

Social Behavior and Children with Autism

Given the complexity of normative social behavior, it is hardly surprising that it is challenging to teach social skills to children with autism who have significant deficits in these areas. Indeed, although deficits and skill sets may vary widely on the spectrum, all children with autism have at least some challenges in social behavior. Some impairment in social function is, after all, a component of the autism diagnosis.

But even in children with autism, social deficits may manifest in many different ways, and with great subtlety (Klin, Jones, Schultz, Volkmar, & Cohen, 2002). It is not uncommon, for example, for a child with autism to initially avoid social interaction all together. For example, one youngster at the Alpine Learning Group abruptly left preferred play activities when a teacher simply sat next to him in the play area. For other children, the deficits in social behavior may be more apparent in their lack of attention to important social cues such as not knowing when a social partner is no longer interested in a topic of conversation. A child with autism who has well-developed vocal verbal behavior skills, for example, may still select inappropriate conversational topics, or dwell on chosen subjects too long. So, too, a child with considerable social motivation may engage in repetitive behavior that is socially stigmatizing, and which limits the extent to which peers are willing to socially interact with him. And a single fundamental skill deficit may also lead to other social impairments: A child who experiences difficulty initiating or sustaining eye contact may struggle to share nonverbal experiences, or to interpret another person's facial expressions.

Thus, while autism by definition involves the impairment of social skills, that impairment presents with as much subtlety and complexity as appropriate social behavior may present in neurotypical persons.

Still, it is widely understood and well documented that children with autism can be taught certain social skills (for reviews see: Gillis & Butler, 2007; Matson, Matson, & Rivet, 2007; White, Koenig, & Scahill, 2007; Reichow & Volkmar, 2010). Using the tools of applied behavior analysis, learners with autism can be taught many of the foundational skills that are the building blocks of social behavior, and practitioners and parents alike may rely on research-based strategies to increase a child's motivation to engage in social activities more consistently and independently. To be sure, the subtleties of social behavior necessitate keen assessment and creative methodology. And, even then, certain social skills may prove elusive, notwithstanding the quality of our interventions. But the success can be palpable, and meaningful: as with social behavior itself, we know it when we see it.

Assessment and Goal Selection

Before one can start teaching socials skills, it's essential to conduct an assessment of the child's social behavior. A number of variables inform assessment and goal selection. Skinner's analysis of verbal behavior (1957) and his conceptualization of the different verbal operants (mand, echoic, tact, intraverbal, and so on) is instructive in helping to identify both social skills to target and potential reinforcing contingencies. For example, when a child points to an item in the environment and says that item's name (e.g., "A plane!"), and is content with his mother's reaction and praise, then that verbal operant is a tact (i.e., a label) maintained by generalized social reinforcers. Thus, when teaching a child to initiate bids for joint attention, it may be necessary to teach the child a sufficient tact repertoire before initiating instruction in the skill itself. Moreover, since tacts are thought to be maintained by generalized social reinforcers, efforts should be made to use these types of rewards for social responses that incorporate tacts, such as bids for joint attention, or comments. In fact, emerging research indicates that these responses can be successfully shaped with social contingencies alone (e.g., see Taylor and Hoch, 2008b).

Similarly, asking questions is an important social skill, but it is also a mand. It is hypothesized that mands are maintained by specific stimuli—in this case, the answer to the question—and occur only when there is sufficient motivation. As such, interventions to teach children to initiate questions incorporate ways to increase a child's motivation to ask the question. Likewise, the instructor ensures that the answer provided is itself reinforcing. For example, when teaching a child to ask, "Where are you going," an adult may abruptly leave a fun interaction (e.g., a pretend birthday party) that she is having with the child. The abrupt disruption increases the likelihood that the child will want to know where the adult is going. The teacher then prompts the child to ask the question, and provides an answer that leads to important information, such as "I'm going to get us some more ice cream!" In this case, the adult is increasing the likelihood that the child will want to know the answer to the question, while at the same time increasing the reinforcing nature of the answer.

Mands may also serve to gain access to tangible items. In this case, teachers can arrange the environment in such a way to increase mands toward others, thereby increasing the rate of initiations toward others. In one study we conducted, we taught children with autism to mand (request) tangible items from peers. Peers were taught to withhold the child's preferred items until the child asked the peer for the items. Over time, the children with autism began to approach their peers more often to ask for the items—one step in the direction of social behavior.

On the other hand, more complex social skills (e.g., conversation) require the learner to discriminate among many different stimuli simultaneously. According to Skinner, intraverbals may place several distinct verbal responses under the control of a single word or group of words, and, in turn, different stimulus words may control the production of a single response. For example, the single comment "I'm going on vacation next week" may be discriminative for several unique responses, such as, "Where are you going?"; "I was on vacation last week"; "You're going to miss Mary's party!" and so on. Thus, complex verbal interactions require an individual to vary his or her responses in relation to many different, shifting variables—no small task for learners with autism. Faced with these instructional challenges, Skinner's analysis of verbal behavior may provide a framework for understanding the potential discriminative stimuli that may occasion responding, as well as the reinforcers that may maintain them. By considering these variables when selecting goals and designing interventions, we may increase the efficiency with which the responses are learned.

Considerations for Assessment

A thorough assessment will lead to identification of potential target goals as well as appropriate instructional methodology. There are a number of published social skills assessments and questionnaires that can assist practitioners in identifying gaps in social skills and targeting objectives. These include The Walker-McConnell Scale of Social Competence and School Adjustment – Elementary version, (1995); The Autism Social Skills Profile (ASSP), 2007; etc. In addition, various published curriculum may point parents and teachers in the direction of specific social skills to target (e.g., Taylor & Jasper, 2001; Weiss & Harris, 2001). In general, though, when a particular assessment tool is not used, social skills are assessed through direct observation, along with parent or teacher interviews, and with consideration of a number of variables:

Developmental Norms: Recognized developmental norms will provide a framework and continuing guide for any assessment. As is widely understood, certain behaviors routinely develop at certain ages. Not surprisingly, teaching interventions are far more effective when educational goals are correlated to appropriate developmental stages. Joint attention, for example, typically develops when a child is 9 to 12 months old. Accordingly, targeting joint attention for a toddler is developmentally appropriate. Alternatively, many theory of mind related responses do not seem to emerge until after age four or five years, so attempts to teach such skills to a toddler would be inappropriate.

Initiations and Responses to Initiations: Attention should be paid not only to a child's responses to the initiations of others (e.g., answering questions presented by a peer), but also to the child's own initiations to others (e.g., asking a peer questions). Because responding and initiating are two different response classes, it cannot be assumed that a child who is able to respond to another's social initiation will also initiate the same responses with others. A recent study on joint attention conducted at Alpine Learning Group illustrates this principle (Taylor & Hoch, 2008a). Although participants in the study learned to respond to bids for joint attention, they did not initiate joint attention bids as a result of learning to respond, indicating that initiation and responses often must be taught separately and specifically.

Nonvocal Behavior: The assessment should also include examination of both vocal verbal behavior (e.g., initiates greetings) and nonvocal behavior (e.g., makes eye contact with listeners). While vocal responses may be the most apparent to an observer, consideration must also be given to the nonvocal responses that emerge independently, those that accompany vocal utterances (e.g., gestures), and to more subtle nonvocal behavior (e.g., sustaining eye contact).

Environmental and Contextual Variables: Social behavior can be highly variable and may be context specific. For example, a child inclined to initiate play in the classroom may not do so on the playground, or a child capable of engaging in conversation with adults may struggle to do so with peers. As a result, assessment includes direct observation of responding in different environments, with different stimuli and with different people.

Social and Cultural Norms: The assessment must also take into account social behaviors or social norms that are more appropriate in certain contexts or cultures than others. For instance, social behavior at work or in a classroom is distinct from social behavior on the playground or in the lunchroom. Similarly, a child's cultural background and social environment may make particular responses more appropriate than others. Ethnic and religious groups often employ different greetings, for example, or have different expectations regarding physical contact. These considerations can be important in determining appropriate learning goals.

Behavioral Challenges: Lastly, the assessment should determine whether the child displays any challenging behavior that may impact or impede the development of social skills and social relationships. For example, if the child engages in high rates of repetitive behavior, such as making loud noises or talking to herself, interventions specifically targeting the problem behavior may be a prerequisite to effectively improving related social skills.

Consideration for Goal Selection

Once a thorough assessment is conducted with consideration of the above variables, teachers prioritize objectives to incorporate into the child's immediate treatment program. The assessment, however, is likely to yield many more programs than can possibly be implemented. For example, at Alpine, it was determined that a newly enrolled student, Billy, did not initiate a vast array of social responses. Among other things, he did not make eye contact when speaking, avoided interactions with peers, and could not answer basic social questions. His teachers were then faced with prioritizing objectives and identifying the most relevant skills to target in his current program—no easy task. Prioritizing objectives, however, can be aided by considering the following:

Age and General Skills: The first is the child's age, and his general skills in other areas. For example, if a child is sixteen months old but does not speak, and actively avoids initiating eye contact with others, it may be most relevant to target initiation of eye contact in order to gain access to a preferred activity, or to concentrate on social turn-taking games that of necessity involve eye contact (e.g., peek-a-boo). On the other hand, for a teenager who demonstrates good vocal verbal behavior and is participating in a community work program, making small talk with coworkers on breaks may be a more immediately pertinent goal. In the example of Billy, despite having a well developed manding (requesting) repertoire, he did not make eye contact when speaking. Since he had certain skills (requesting) but lacked other skills (eye contact), which impeded the social nature of the interaction, it was determined that targeting eye contact when speaking would be an appropriate goal.

Environment-Appropriate Goals: Second, consideration should be given to the social skills that are needed or required within the environments that make up the student's social and educational world. For example, if the child is attending a typical preschool environment, increasing both interest in peers and initiations toward peers may be a priority (Taylor & Jasper, 2001). By the same token, if a child is poised to begin attending a community recreation program, learning to wait his turn to engage in an activity may be an appropriate social goal. Although Billy was primarily going to be attending school at Alpine, the environment is one that values eye contact. Therefore, the skill would likely be required and reinforced within his immediate school environment and was relevant to target in his immediate program.

Family Priorities: Third, it is important to examine parent or care provider priorities: what is important for the family? For example, parents may be interested in having their child interact with siblings, participate in community or religious activities, report on their daily activities, or participate in a family dinner. Or a sibling may want the child to learn how to play a particular game. Not surprisingly, families are highly motivated to assist in teaching or generalizing skills when they are actively involved in selecting the targets that matter most to them. In the case of Billy, his parents were very interested in having him answer questions presented by community and family members. As a result, we prioritized teaching Billy to answer basic social questions such as where he attended school, his favorite subjects, and his preferred leisure activities. These responses were highly valued by his parents and were readily integrated into community and family interactions.

Ease of Acquisition and Range of Application: Fourth, when possible, goals are identified that: 1) may be learned with relative ease, and 2) will have the biggest impact across a wide variety of environments and people. For example, responding to greetings will affect the learner's interactions at school, at home, in the community, and at work. Likewise, the skill will be used in interactions with peers, family members, coworkers, customers, and community members alike. In the same way, it may make sense to prioritize a simpler skill with broad application—say, answering social questions—before focusing on more challenging skills, such as interpreting facial expressions. For Billy, the social questions he was learning were highly valued by his parents and had a broad range of application (e.g., at parties, with relatives, in the community, etc.). But our decision to teach this skill was also informed by the fact that Billy was able to imitate vocal responses fairly well. This indicated to us that he would learn the skill of answering questions with relative ease.

Individual Interests: Sometimes specific skills actually lend themselves to a learner's existing interests. At Alpine Learning Group, for example, one student who was fond of video games never included others in his play activities. Rather than teach him to participate in group sports or board games, instructors first concentrated on teaching him to play video games with friends and peers, rather than alone. Likewise, if a student struggles to initiate and maintain conversation with others, we may first teach her to talk about her favorite topics, and address the appropriateness and variety of conversation topics later. In unusual cases, sophisticated learners with autism may even help identify their own learning targets. Whatever the case, individual interests may be useful both in selecting goals and implementing interventions.

Flexibility in Sequencing: In the best of all worlds, the development of social skills would follow along a continuum, beginning with early social responses such as eye contact and joint attention, then building incrementally to more complex behaviors, such as inferring another's intentions or attitudes and responding accordingly. Because children with autism present with such complex learning challenges and uneven skills across many areas, however, social skills instruction rarely follows a typical, linear sequence. For example, an assessment might identify that a fairly challenged teenager with autism has not yet developed many early social responses, such as joint attention or the ability to read facial expressions. Given his age and learning challenges, however, it may not be appropriate to target these early social skills, but rather to concentrate on responding to greetings and saying, "Excuse me" when someone is in his way. In other words, the selection of goals is informed by learner characteristics and the functionality of the social skill that is identified. While consideration of necessary prerequisite skills is essential, goal selection does not necessarily follow a strict sequence.

Teaching Social Skills

The Role of Motivation

The consequences used to shape behavior are a core component of any intervention targeting social skills. In the early development of neurotypical children, certain social responses appear to be shaped by social reinforcers alone. These social reinforcers are consequences delivered by another person or persons, and they may take several forms: facial expressions (e.g., smiles), vocalizations (e.g., "What a big boy!"), gestures (e.g., clapping), physical interactions (e.g., affection, tickles), or any combination thereof. Children with autism, and particularly those who happen to be significantly socially avoidant, often struggle to appreciate these types of social reinforcers. As a result, early in treatment, it is often difficult to shape the social behavior of children with autism using social engagement alone, and it is sometimes necessary to devote time to developing the reinforcing potential of social engagement and interaction. While applied research is much needed in this area, there are several clinical strategies that may increase a child's interest in social interaction:

Pairing Social Engagement with Preferred Tangible Items or Activities: As a first step, social engagement may be paired with tangible reinforcers to encourage the student to appreciate the social consequences alongside the tangible reward. Over time, the tangible items may be gradually removed, until only the social stimuli remain. Take, as an example, a young preschooler who was extremely avoidant of both adults and other children, to the extent that she refused to open her eyes in the presence of others, and threw a tantrum when faced with almost any social interaction. Nevertheless, because her favorite activity was watching videos, Alpine Learning Group instructors began pairing teachers with access to preferred videos. Initially, the teacher simply sat in the room behind the child when the video played. Gradually, the teacher moved closer and closer to the student. Over time, access to the video was paired with physical contact (e.g., patting her back and stroking her hair) and positive comments.

In time, the teacher was able to interact with the child before turning on the video, and finally, without turning the video on at all. In the end, the child began to approach the teacher on her own and initiate the interactions (e.g., extending her arms to be picked up, asking for tickles, etc.). Teachers were then able to introduce social engagement and interaction as reinforcers in her other learning activities. Emerging research likewise supports the proposition that providing social interactions along with the child's requested activity can lead to increases in social engagement (Koegel, Vernon & Koegel, 2009).

Providing Preferred Activities Noncontingently Alongside Social Engagement: Initially, to strengthen the adult presence as a reinforcer, teachers may provide a child's highly preferred items or activities noncontingently (freely, without requiring the child to work for them) along with social interaction, with the goal of conditioning the adult as a potential reinforcer. When adults become conditioned reinforcers, it may increase the likelihood that the child will approach and interact with the adult, both when the preferred item or activity is present, and afterwards, when it has been faded or removed. The peers in Alpine Learning Group's peer modeling program, for example, are taught to provide activities noncontingently to the child with autism, which, in turn, increases the learner's interest in the peers (Taylor & Jasper, 2001). One youngster, for instance, rarely approached peers and did not request activities from them even though he had learned to request items from adults. Alpine staff devised a program of having the peers provide preferred toys to the child on a fixed schedule (e.g., every five minutes). Over time, the child with autism began to approach his peers more consistently and started to request items that the peers held in view.

Using Social Interaction to Improve the Value of a Preferred Item or Activity: Another strategy is to have an adult use social interaction to improve the value of a preferred item or activity. Imagine a child who already enjoys spinning around on an office chair. If an adult can help the child spin faster and longer, thereby intensifying the experience, the child may begin to appreciate these interactions with adults and seek them out more regularly. One child, for example, liked to jump on the trampoline but whined and cried if someone tried to jump with her. Her teachers started by holding her hands and helping her to jump higher. Eventually, the child started to pull her teachers toward the trampoline. While the initiation may initially have been to have the teacher help her jump higher, attainment of the desired response (jumping higher) was dependent on social contact with another (holding her teacher by the hand and leading her to the trampoline).

Variables That Affect Motivation

The demonstration of a social skill will also be directly related to the degree to which the individual is "motivated" to engage in the response. Tom, for example, may successfully learn *how* to initiate a conversation with friends at school but continue to remain otherwise disinterested in peer interaction, playing predominantly by himself. A child such as Tom may choose not to engage in a particular social response despite the opportunity and ability to do so. In this example, we may say that Tom lacks motivation to engage in the social interaction.

Motivation is a complex concept, in which reinforcer effectiveness is influenced by a host of different variables, including the rate, quality, and magnitude of the reinforcers; delay to reinforcers; and the response effort to obtain the reinforcer (Davison & McCarthy, 1988). Consider, for example, the factors that might, on any given night, influence your decision to either go to a movie with friends or to stay home alone. You may consider how far you have to drive to get to the movie or how draining your work week was (i.e., response effort), which friends have asked and whether they are seeing a comedy or a horror movie (i.e., quality of the reinforcer), and whether they are seeing an early show or a late show (i.e., delay to the reinforcer). And while one factor may be the deciding one in your evaluation, it is equally possible that your ultimate decision may depend on an interaction of several, if not all, of the factors.

For someone with autism, social responding will be related to the same sorts of variables. For example, if Johnny has to wait until he gets home before he earns his reward for being social on the playground at school, the delay to accessing reinforcers may be too great, and may impede the response. Or, if the requirement to earn a tangible reward involves numerous challenging social responses simultaneously (e.g., initiate to five friends, avoid specific topics in conversation, stand at appropriate distance, make eye contact, etc.), the effort to obtain the reinforcer may likewise be too great. Faced with either scenario, a child with autism may choose not to engage in the targeted social behavior.

The potential impact of motivation on responding should not be underestimated, and clinicians must carefully and systematically consider, and regularly evaluate, how motivational variables affect social responding in particular (Hoch, McComas, Johnson, Guenther, & Faranda, 2002). Some practical applications and considerations may include:

- Are the reinforcers for social responding delivered at a sufficiently high rate? For example, if the student receives points for initiating play statements, are points being provided frequently enough?
- Is the reinforcer of sufficient quality? For example, when teaching a new social skill, is a better or bigger reward being used, one that is qualitatively better than rewards being used for other responses (e.g., using ice cream instead of a sip of juice)?
- Is the delay between the response and the reinforcer appropriate? For example, is the child required to initiate conversation with peers during recess and then have to wait until the end of the school day to receive praise and a reward?
- Does the social skill take too much effort, requiring too many responses simultaneously for the child to earn a reward? For

example, is the child expected to initiate conversation, track the person's facial expression to assess interest, make appropriate shifts in topic, *and* stand at the appropriate distance? Several responses that are individually manageable may together become unwieldy and too effortful for the available reinforcer.

Motivation Operations

In addition to the variables that can influence the effectiveness of a stimulus as a reinforcer, a learner's motivation to engage in a social behavior will be affected by Motivating Operations (MO) such as deprivation and satiation (Michael, 1993).

MOs alter the effectiveness of reinforcers or punishers, and, as a result, alter the frequency of specific responses related to those consequences. For example, if someone is sufficiently deprived of fluids and as a result is thirsty, they are more likely to engage in a response in order to obtain a drink (e.g., enter a store and purchase a bottle of water). Imagine how this might relate to social behavior. While doing yard work one morning, you greet your neighbor, who proceeds to tell you a long story about a vacation he just took. Later that day, you spot your neighbor in aisle three of the local market, and quickly turn down aisle two to avoid another episode of "small talk." In this example, "too much" social interaction with your neighbor that morning has decreased the likelihood that you will head down aisle three to initiate a greeting. You might be more likely to approach your neighbor and initiate a chat had it been a while since your last encounter.

In the same way, learners with autism will be influenced by general states of deprivation and satiation with regard to various stimuli. For example, a student is more likely to initiate play with a friend who is playing with one of his preferred toys if he has not recently enjoyed access to the toy.

From a practical and strategic standpoint, one can contrive motivating operations in order to increase a learner's motivation to engage in particular forms of social interaction (Sundberg, Loeb, Hale, & Eigenheer, 2002; Taylor, Hoch, Potter, Rodriguez, Spinnato, & Kalaigian, 2005). Consider the following:

- Try restricting access to certain preferred items, withholding them for use as rewards only when teaching the target social skill.
- Provide the learner with a preferred activity (e.g., a farm set), but remove a piece or item necessary to fully engage in the activity; then, teach the student to ask a peer for the missing item.
- Provide the learner with a toy that he enjoys but is unable to operate on his own (e.g., a mechanical top that spins); then, teach him to ask a peer for assistance in order to get the toy to work.

- Hide items necessary to complete a task, and teach the student to approach another person to ask where the items are.
- Place preferred toys in areas the child cannot reach, and teach him to ask a friend for help in retrieving the items.
- During snack time, have a peer control access to the child's preferred snack items, and teach the child to ask the peer for the snack.
- Give the student an activity that requires multiple pieces to complete (e.g., a puzzle), and have a peer control access to the items. Then, teach the child to ask the peer for each item to complete the task.

Specific Interventions

In addition to considering how to increase motivation, before beginning instruction, the teacher identifies a prompt that can reliably produce the social response. For example, if a child is being taught to say "Hi" when walking by someone in the hallway, the teacher would determine whether the student can imitate the word "Hi." If so, the prompt is used to teach the student to respond in the presence of the more relevant discriminative stimulus (e.g., the presence of someone walking by in the hallway). Because the goal is to teach the learner to respond in the presence of the relevant stimulus, and not merely to imitate the target phrase, the teacher removes or "fades" her model of the response "Hi" so that the child initiates the greeting when approaching the person in the hallway rather than waiting to be prompted. There are a number of strategies outlined in the literature to promote responses and to fade and remove prompts over time.

Errorless Teaching: Time Delay and Most to Least Prompting Procedures

A common prompting strategy is a *progressive time delay.* In this technique, the instructor provides the prompt (e.g., a vocal model of the greeting) immediately upon the appearance or presentation of the relevant stimulus (e.g., the person the student is expected to greet). This procedure is repeated until the learner imitates the vocal model consistently in the presence of the relevant stimulus (the person whom he is greeting). Next, the instructor gradually increases the time—say, in two-second increments—between the presentation of the relevant stimulus (the presence of the person to greet) and the prompt (the teacher's vocal model). Once the learner can respond reliably with a significant delay (e.g., six or more seconds), the prompt may be removed entirely. Time delay procedures have been shown to be effective in teaching a number of socially relevant responses, including statements of affection (Charlop & Walsh, 1986), and question-asking (Taylor & Harris, 1995).

Another strategy is *"most to least prompting,"* which involves systematically presenting less and less of the original vocal model. In our greeting example, an instructor transferring stimulus control by most to least prompting would slowly delete the final syllables or sounds of the prompt. In the case of "Hello," the instructor would begin with the complete prompt, then shift to "Hell-," "He-," and finally "Hhh-." As a final step, any remaining vestige of the prompt should be removed, so that the child produces the response "Hello!" without the instructor providing any portion of the model.

Time delay and most to least prompting procedures may be particularly beneficial in the early stages of a student's learning process, as they systematically reduce errors and increase opportunities for a child to produce a correct response that the instructor may reinforce accordingly. At the same time, though, these procedures may lead to reliance on adults to initiate responses, particularly if the teacher has not effectively faded or removed prompts. The strategies listed below may increase independence because they reduce reliance directly on adults to initiate responses.

Script Fading Procedures

A script is a written word, phrase, or sentence that prompts a learner with autism to say or do specific responses in certain contexts. Imagine, for example, that Jane's mom places in her daughter's lunch bag a card with the written text, "Today my mom made me a sandwich for lunch." At lunchtime, Jane's teacher prompts Jane to take out the card, turn toward a peer, and read aloud the statement on the card. In time, and without any additional prompts from her teacher, Jane may independently remove the card from her lunch bag and read the comment to her friend. In this case, the written text prompts Jane's comment, and the textual card has become a discriminative stimulus for the initiation of conversation toward a peer. Once Jane reliably and independently uses the script on the card to initiate the response, her mother would fade the script by removing portions of the text until the card was blank, and Jane was able to comment about what her mother made her for lunch when she removed her lunch from her bag.

A number of studies have documented that script fading may be useful in teaching such social responses as conversational statements to peers (Charlop-Christy & Kelso, 2003), attention gaining statements (Krantz & Mc-Clannahan, 1998), and comments about preferred snacks and leisure activities (Sarakoff, Taylor, & Poulson, 2001).

Audio-taped Scripts

Several studies document the benefits of using audiotaped scripts (Wichnick, Vener, Pyrtek, & Poulson, 2010). An audiotaped script is a recorded vocalization that is used to cue a child to make comments in certain contexts. Consider this example: When Brian is presented with a statement such as "I'm going somewhere," his mother would like him to respond by asking, "Where are you going?" To help him learn this response, Brian's mother could record the target response on an audio device. During teaching sessions, Brian's mother would then present the statement "I'm going somewhere," and immediately activate the recording device so that her son can hear the model and imitate the question. Across successive teaching sessions, Brian's mom would then fade the audiotaped model—like a textual script—from the last to first word, until Brian independently asks the question when presented with his mother's statement.

Of course, audiotaped models closely parallel "live" vocal models. There are, however, important distinctions. For one, audiotaped prompts, by totally removing the risk of human error, provide a consistency in content and inflection that is difficult, if not impossible, to achieve in an instructional program involving numerous teachers and participants. Likewise, audiotaped prompts may be faded without concern for human error or variations in inflection and tone. Moreover, learners using audio prompts may find it easier to distinguish the prompt from the natural discriminative stimulus. After all, a child learning to imitate either verbal or audiotaped responses must learn to discriminate between the stimulus that prompts his response—in our example, the mother's announcement that she is leaving—and the verbal stimulus he should imitate—"Where are you going?" In most cases, learners with autism more readily distinguish between the live and recorded statements, and thus between the stimulus and the modeled response.

Incidental Teaching

Incidental teaching involves arranging the teaching environment in order to increase the initiations of the child with autism toward others in his or her immediate surroundings (Pierce & Schreibman, 1995). For example, a teacher may take all of the child's preferred items and place them on a high shelf, or the teacher may have a peer hold access to a child's preferred items. These intentional environmental modifications increase the likelihood of the child seeking out an adult or peer in order to access these items.

When the child initiates interest in the item or activity, the adult or peer uses the initiation as an opportunity to prompt a response of the child with autism. The item or activity the child has initiated toward is then used as the reinforcer for that response. For example, a teacher may place a child's preferred items in view but out of reach; then, when the child shows an interest in the item, the teacher provides a prompt (e.g., a model) for a social comment about the activity (e.g., "Those are my favorite!" or "Do you want to play that video game with me?"). When the child imitates the model, the child is then provided with the activity and the child and teacher play together. Incidental teaching has the benefit of capitalizing on the child's apparent interests, thereby increasing his motivation to engage in the targeted responses.

Video Modeling Procedures

Video modeling procedures can be used to teach children a variety of socially related responses such as conversational skills (Taylor, Levin, & Jasper, 1999), social initiation skills, giving compliments, and making comments during play activities (MacDonald et al., 2005). Video modeling provides both a vocal and motor model for the child to imitate. For example, when teaching a child with autism and his peer to make statements related to a block building activity, a teacher might create a video of two adults building with blocks and making relevant observations about their shared activity (e.g., "Let's build a skyscraper!"). After watching the videotaped sequence several times, the child is provided with the same building materials used in the video. If the child has the prerequisite skills, he may initiate some of the vocal responses and actions that he viewed in the videotape. There are several variations of video modeling procedures in the literature, including the type of model, the frequency of viewing, and incorporation of reinforcers to shape imitative responses.

Pager Prompts

Pager prompts are vibrating pagers that serve as prompts for the child with autism to produce social responses (Taylor & Levin, 1998). Pager prompts permit instructors to deliver prompts from remote locations, without calling undue attention to the learner. Because they are inconspicuous and unobtrusive, pager prompts are a particularly apt method of teaching in contexts when traditional prompting methods might be socially stigmatizing.

At Alpine Learning Group, we use manually cued pagers which instructors can signal, at their discretion, when specific discriminative stimuli (e.g., a peer) are present, and a motivating operation in effect (e.g., the child picks up a novel toy). In this way, a student can be prompted to respond to a social opportunity by a distant observing teacher. Anecdotal reports suggest that this procedure may be more effective in producing sustained levels of initiations even in the absence of the pager, because the pager's prompt has been specifically paired with the natural stimuli that should occasion the social response.

Selection of Interventions

When initiating social skills instruction, interventions are generally matched both to the skill level of the child with autism and to the specific skill targeted. It may be the case, for example, that certain skills such as answering social questions are most effectively taught in a structured format using discrete trial instruction, particularly if the student is an early learner who requires a good deal of repetition to master skills. In contrast, a child who is able to attend to and discriminate multiple stimuli simultaneously may be taught to initiate bids for joint attention in a play area where there are a wide variety of stimuli available. Thus, social skills interventions are individualized for each child, and often multiple interventions may be employed simultaneously with a given learner—depending on what is being taught. In other words, a child may be learning to answer questions with a discrete trial teaching format, while at the same time learning to initiate eye contact during incidental teaching activities. Thus, a number of factors are considered when choosing an intervention.

The Targeted Skill: Some interventions will lend themselves better to instruction of specific skills. For example, more structured interventions such as discrete trial teaching are beneficial for teaching component skills associated with more complex social behavior, such as answering questions, asking questions, or labeling emotions.

Prior Learning History and Responsiveness to the Intervention: If, for example, you are teaching an adult with autism to initiate greetings while at a worksite, it may be appropriate to use a textual script if the student has well-developed reading skills. If, on the other hand, the student cannot read, modeling or using an audiotaped script will be a more appropriate and effective intervention.

Context: Some interventions will be better suited for use in specific contexts. For example, in-vivo guidance and verbal prompts, even if effective in helping a preschooler with autism to learn to initiate toward peers in a typical preschool class, may prove socially stigmatizing in that context. The same types of prompts (e.g., in-vivo guidance and verbal prompts), however, may be entirely appropriate in an intervention aimed at increasing play statements with siblings at home.

Research Support for the Intervention: Empirical evidence often provides more support for using a given intervention to address a specific social skill, rather than another. For example, there is considerable empirical support demonstrating the efficacy of using textual scripts to teach scripted conversational statements. Likewise, research has established that video modeling is a particularly effective way to teach play-related statements to children with autism (for a review of interventions see Matson, Matson, & Rivet, 2007).

Generalization

Because children with autism have difficulty generalizing skills to novel settings, people, or stimuli, interventions should incorporate procedures to enhance the likelihood of generalization from the outset (Stokes & Bear, 1977). For example, when teaching a child to comment about toys, a variety of toys may be used to prevent repetition of comments about the same toys. Similarly, a variety of people may be used to teach the targeted skills to promote the child's responding across different people. It is likewise important to practice skills in different settings to enhance responding across environments and in the face of environmental changes. Thus, after initially teaching the targeted skills in the school environment, instructors may invite parents to help their child practice the skill at school before instruction proceeds to the student's home.

In some cases, instruction may first involve a specific set of stimuli, and only later will teachers incorporate procedures to enhance generalization. For example, when teaching a more challenged learner how to answer social questions, instructors may begin by asking the question in a specific way (e.g., "What is your name?"), rather than varying the form or content of the question from the start (e.g., "Who are you?" "And you are?", etc.). Over time, instructors introduce variations on the question while still expecting the same response. Similarly, when working with a young learner, a single response (e.g., "John") may initially be taught, and additional responses (e.g., "I'm John," "My name is John," "John Smith," etc.) are introduced over time. Additionally, in some cases, the assessment of generalization occurs with novel stimuli periodically during instruction. Thus, a child may be taught to initiate greetings in the hallway at school, and tests for generalization occur in other locations—the bus, the playground, or the lobby of the child's apartment building, for example.

Data Collection and Analyses

Data on social behavior are collected and analyzed to ensure that interventions are leading to desired changes in response. These may include changes in rate or frequency of responding within a period of time (e.g., the rate per minute of comments toward peers), the duration of a response (e.g., the duration of sustained play with parent), or the percentage of a particular response (e.g., the percentage of correct answers to social questions presented by a peer).

Data may also be recorded on the responding of typically developing peers as a way to determine age-appropriate and socially meaningful learning goals for the child with autism. For example, when designing an intervention to help the child increase the initiation of questions toward peers in a classroom, data are recorded on a typical peer's behavior in the same classroom to arrive at a reasonable goal for the child with autism. Baseline data are also recorded on the child with autism in order to correlate his actual skill level with the data on typically developing peers. The relationship of these two measures allows us to set a teaching goal that reflects both the child's ability and socially meaningful expectations.

Data collection and analyses are also ongoing components of a successful intervention. It is not always easy, however, to collect data on social behavior while simultaneously working to shape and transform that behavior. Imagine, for example, teaching a child to engage in conversation with a peer while also prompting her to make appropriate remarks, sustain eye contact, and respond to the peer's comments, all while taking data on the student's responses. Juggling so many tasks would be a challenge and likely to interfere with instruction. In such circumstances, teaching may take place across several sessions and a probe session is then conducted without prompts and reinforcers to assess performance.

Fortunately, technological innovations may be available to facilitate data collection. For example, it is now possible to videotape teaching sessions using a small, unobtrusive recording device, and to then review and record the data later. Similarly, computerized data recording programs and applications designed for handheld devices such as smart phones may make data collection more efficient, discreet, and portable.

Social Validity

As we've learned, social behavior is a complex phenomenon, but one which, using the techniques of applied behavior, may be conceptualized and taught to individuals who lack such skills. And while the outcome of our interventions may be assessed using a variety of scientific measures, the true success of our teaching lies in its benefit to the individuals, families, and communities we serve. This means that in some cases, promising data may not necessarily represent a successful result. We may be able to teach a child with autism to initiate interactions with typically developing peers, but the initiations may fail if the peers do not view the responses we have taught as rewarding or meaningful. Peers are unlikely to reinforce such initiations, and ultimately the child with autism will fail to respond at all.

In the same sense, we may subsequently discover that our interventions have taught skills that lack an essential quality, and that the lack undermines their social meaning. For example, you may be able to teach a child to respond to someone's injury with a concerned statement such as "Are you all right?" but if the child does not make the statement with the proper intonation, the concerned message may be lost.

Thus, in social contexts it becomes particularly important to assess the social validity of our teaching outcomes. This may include weighing parents' or family members' opinion of the meaningfulness or functionality of the skills prior to teaching, or evaluating the skills once they are demonstrated. Social validity may also be assessed by soliciting community members to view video footage of a child's skills both before and after the teaching intervention. For example, instructors may ask a parent or sibling to watch videos of a baseline probe and then sessions conducted after the student has attained mastery of the target skill, and then to discuss the positive social changes, if any, they notice in comparing the two sequences.

Assessments of social validity may also be informal. For example, at Alpine Learning Group, adults with autism are employed in community-based worksites. In order to identify relevant learning targets, staff members observe social behavior common to the work environment and identify relevant objectives based on that context. Staff may also ask the individual's supervisors to share their impression of a skill once it has been taught: whether it is meaningful, how the skill might be improved, or whether another skill seems a more important target. Similarly, peers may be asked to rate or gauge the social behavior of a child after he has mastered the targeted skills. For example, for children who participate in inclusive educational environments, peers may be asked to provide their impressions of the child's social skills within specific contexts (e.g., "Do you like the games that Jane can play?").

Because social behavior involves complex interactions among many different responses (e.g., what is said, how it is said, and to whom it is said, etc.), seeking out independent evaluations of learned responses from several sources is essential in assessing the efficacy of our teaching interventions.

This information is indispensible, for although the dynamic fabric of our social community sets the occasion for teachers and behavior analysts to improve the social behavior of those in our care, it is our students' progress and skilled responding that reinforces our continued work in this area.

References

Charlop-Christy, M. H., & Kelso, S. E. (2003). Teaching children with autism conversational speech using a cue card/written script program. *Education & Treatment of Children, 26,* 108-127.

Davison, M., & McCarthy, D. (1988). *The matching law: A research review.* Hillsdale, NJ: Earlbaum.

Gillis, J. M., & Butler, R. (2007). Social skills intervention for preschoolers with autism spectrum disorder: A description of single-subject design studies. *Journal of Early Intensive Behavioral Intervention, 2,* 532-546.

Hoch, H., McComas, J., Johnson, L., Faranda, N., & Guenther, S. L. (2002). The effects of magnitude and quality of reinforcement on choice responding during play activities. *Journal of Applied Behavior Analysis, 35,* 171-182.

Klin, A., Jones, W., Schultz, R., Volkmar, F., & Cohen, D. (2002). Defining and quantifying the social phenotype in autism. *American Journal of Psychiatry, 159,* 895-908.

Koegel, R. L., Vernon, T. W., & Koegel, L. K. (2009). Improving social initiations in young children with autism using reinforcers with embedded social interactions. *Journal of Autism and Developmental Disorders, 39,* 1240-1251.

Krantz, P. J., & McClannahan, L .E. (1993). Teaching children with autism to initiate to peers: Effects of a script fading procedure. *Journal of Applied Behavior Analysis, 26,* 121-132.

Krantz, P. J., & McClannahan, L. E. (1998). Social interaction skills for children with autism: A script-fading procedure for beginning readers. *Journal of Applied Behavior Analysis, 31,* 191-202.

MacDonald, R. P. F., Clark, M., Garrigan, E., & Vangala, M. (2005). Using video modeling to teach pretend play to children with autism. *Behavioral Interventions, 20,* 225-238.

Matson, J. L., Matson, M. L., & Rivet, T. T. (2007). Social-skills treatments for children with autism spectrum disorders: An overview. *Behavior Modification, 31,* 682-707.

McClannahan, L. E., & Krantz, P. J. (2005). *Teaching conversation to children with autism: Scripts and script fading.* Bethesda, MD: Woodbine House.

Michael, J. (1993). Establishing operations. *The Behavior Analyst, 16,* 191-206.

Pierce, K., & Schreibman, L.(1995). Increasing complex social behaviors in children with autism: Effects of a peer mediated pivotal response training. *Journal of Applied Behavior Analysis, 28,* 285-295.

Reichow, B., & Volkmar, F. R. (2010). Social skills intervention for individuals with autism: Evaluation for evidence-based practices within a best evidence synthesis framework. *Journal of Autism and Developmental Disorders, 40*, 149-166.

Romanczyk, R. G., White, S. J., & Gillis, J. M. (2005). Social skills vs. skilled social behavior: A problematic distinction in autism spectrum disorders. *Journal of Early and Intensive Behavior Intervention, 2*, 177-193.

Sarakoff, R. A., Taylor, B. A., & Poulson, C. L. (2001). Teaching children with autism to engage in conversational exchanges: Script-fading with embedded textual stimuli. *Journal of Applied Behavior Analysis, 31,* 81-84.

Skinner, B. F. (1975). *Verbal behavior.* New York, NY: Appleton Century Crofts.

Skinner, B. F. (1953). *Science and human behavior.* New York, NY: The Free Press.

Stokes, T. F., & Baer, D. M. (1977). An implicit technology of generalization. *Journal of Applied Behavior Analysis, 10*, 349-367.

Sundberg, M. L., Loeb, M., Hale, L., & Eigenheer, P. (2002). Contriving establishing operations to teach mands for information. *The Analysis of Verbal Behavior, 18*, 14-28.

Taylor, B. A. (2001). Teaching Peer Social Skills to Children with Autism. In C. Maurice, G. Green, & R. Fox (Eds.), *Making a difference: Behavioral intervention in autism.* Austin, TX: Pro-Ed.

Taylor, B. A., & Harris, S. (1995). Teaching children with autism to seek information: Acquisition of novel information and generalization of responding. *Journal of Applied Behavior Analysis, 28*, 3-14.

Taylor, B. A., & Hoch, H. (2008a). Facilitating language in learners with autism: Stimulus control technology. In P. Sturmey, & A. Fitzer (Eds.), *Applied behavior analysis and language acquisition in people with autism spectrum disorders.* Austin, TX: Pro-Ed.

Taylor, B. A., & Hoch, H. (2008b). Teaching children with autism to respond to and to initiate bids for joint attention. *Journal of Applied Behavior Analysis, 41,* 377-391.

Taylor, B. A., Hoch, H., & Potter, B. (2005). Manipulating establishing operations to promote initiations toward peers in children with autism. *Research in Developmental Disabilities, 26*, 385-392.

Taylor, B. A., & Jasper S. (2001). Teaching programs and activities to improve the social behavior of children with autism. In C. Maurice, G. Green, & R. Fox (Eds.), *Making a difference: Behavioral intervention in autism.* Austin, TX: Pro-Ed.

Taylor, B. A., & Levin, L. (1998). Teaching a student with autism to make verbal initiations: Effects of a tactile prompt. *Journal of Applied Behavior Analysis, 31,* 651-654.

Taylor, B. A., Levin, L., & Jasper, S. (1999). Increasing play-related statements in children with autism toward their siblings: Effects of video modeling. *Journal of Developmental and Physical Disabilities, 11*, 253-264.

Thiemann, K. S., & Goldstein, H. (2004). Effects of peer training and written text cueing on social communication of school-age children with pervasive developmental disorder. *Journal of Speech, Language, and Hearing Research, 47,* 126-144.

Weiss, M. J., & Harris, S. L. (2001). *Reaching out, joining in: Teaching social skills to young children with autism.* Bethesda, MD: Woodbine House.

Wert, B. Y., & Neisworth, J. T. (2003). Effects of video self-modeling on spontaneous requesting in children with autism. *Journal of Positive Behavior Interventions, 5,* 30-34.

White, S. W., Keonig, K., & Scahill, L. (2007). Social skills development in children with autism spectrum disorders: A review of the intervention research. *Journal of Autism and Developmental Disorders, 37,* 1858-1868.

Wichnick, A. M., Vener, S. M., Pyrtek, M., & Poulson, C. (2010). The effect of a script-fading procedure on responses to peer initiations among young children with autism. *Research in Autism Spectrum Disorders, 4,* 290-299.

2

Sunny Starts
DANCE Instruction for Parents and Toddlers with ASD

Shahla Ala'i -Rosales, Samantha Cermak,
and Kristín Guðmundsdóttir

Typical toddlers and their parents engage in a graceful "social dance." In a longitudinal study of 42 families, Hart and Risley (1995/1999) described the social and linguistic interactions of parents and their typically developing children. They observed infants growing into toddlerhood for an hour once per month over the course of two and a half years. Then they quantitatively and qualitatively offered insights into the complex and beautiful "social dance" that takes place between toddlers and parents. The researchers characterized the interactions as occurring in frequent, discontinuous episodes; with both parents and toddlers engaging in leading and following behaviors; both partners enticing or prolonging interactions; and, perhaps most importantly, parents and toddlers often appearing to stay together for no other reason than enjoyment of the social interaction itself.

Unfortunately the "social dance" that takes place between toddlers with autism and their parents is, at best, awkward, and, at worst, heartbreaking. Both dance partners face challenges. By definition, children with autism do not respond to the social world in the same way as children without a diagnosis of autism. They have difficulty communicating to partners, and they are not interested in the same activities and events as their interaction partners (American Psychiatric Association, 2000). The situation is exacerbated by the fact that parents of very newly diagnosed toddlers face a myriad of concerns and stressors associated with their child's disorder that could affect overall interaction patterns. Furthermore, the child's lack of social relatedness has been associated with overall parenting stress. There is, however, indication that parent training can alleviate some of that stress and increase the quality of interactions for both partners (e.g., Brookman-Frazee, 2004).

Parent training has been offered as both a means to increase child skills and to directly address the quality of parent-child relationships (see Marcus, Kunce, & Scholper, 2005). For example, training programs have taught parents to increase their children's communication skills, to increase imitation and play skills, to increase parental encouragement of positive sibling interactions, and to increase parental responsiveness. Furthermore, a growing number of studies have focused specifically on parent-toddler interventions.

Sunny Starts is a parent-training program that was created to help families improve their "social dance." The program is part of the Department of Behavior Analysis at the University of North Texas, and offers services in the local community, at Easter Seals North Texas, a nonprofit agency serving people with disabilities. Sunny Starts is also a service-learning program (Hartman, 1999), designed to provide the local community benefit while, at the same time, teaching graduate students to effectively and compassionately implement interventions, training, and research.

The purpose of this chapter is to describe Sunny Starts as it relates to the development of social skills in very young children with autism. In this chapter we will explain our views of social behavior and our basic working assumptions when approaching interventions for toddlers and parents. We will then describe the sequence of the program, including assessment and data collection procedures, our teaching and training methods, and our approaches to generalization. Finally, we will describe some family experiences in our program. The families have given permission for us to do so; however, many details will be changed in order to protect their privacy.

Defining Social Behavior

In the broadest sense, we view social behavior as any interaction that occurs between two people. There are competent ways of interacting that lead to progressive, productive, and fulfilling relationships in life; in fact, social competence is considered "a central organizing theme" for all human development (Odom, McConnel, & McEvoy, 1992). There are also ways of interacting that lead to limited or arrested development. One of the primary reasons a child receives a diagnosis with autism has to do with the way he or she interacts (or doesn't interact) with people (American Psychiatric Association, 2000).

Limited social competence is deemed the most challenging aspect of autism, and, for this reason, social skills training for children is considered one of the most robust, albeit difficult, areas of intervention research. Most of this social skills research is with preschool and school-aged children and involves chronological peers. The interventions have typically aimed to increase skills thought to contribute to social competence (e.g., sharing, conversations, co-operative play) and the measures of success have included increases in the overall initiations, responses, and interactions (McConnell, 2002).

In the case of Sunny Starts, we work with the toddler's main social part-ners, his or her parents. We view their interactions as a starting point for all later social interactions. We are interested in teaching behaviors that improve family interactions and show some promise for promoting later social devel-opment and relationships.

The social behaviors we target for intervention are relatively simple. The context and the meaning of the behaviors are derived from the effects that "social" responses have on others. The effect is, to some degree, more im-portant than the behaviors themselves. This viewpoint is sometimes referred to as "contextualistic behavior analysis" (Haring, 1992). This approach is in keeping with B.F. Skinner's functional approach to verbal and social behav-ior and takes into account the motivational functions of behavior as well as contextual stimulus control (Skinner, 1953). Within such an account, "social skills" such as a toddler gazing with a smile at his father, who responds with tickles and a lively song, can be understood within a context:

> *The skill has to be understood in relation to the goals that a*
> *child has for his or her social behavior, the quality of support*
> *that the social behavior receives from others, and the power of*
> *the simple presence and responsiveness of others in the child's*
> *natural settings to increase the occurrence of the behavior. In*
> *other words, a more contextualistic analysis considers the goals*
> *and functions of the behavior from the child's perspective, as well*
> *as the social responses that the child receives in interactions with*
> *others, which reinforces social behavior (Haring, 1992, 309).*

In the Sunny Starts program, we look at the child's goals and effects as well as the parent's goals and effects. The primary concern is with the back and forth rhythm, the dance, between the interaction partners: Can we facili-tate an increased number of initiations and responses? How can we help the partners prolong those interactions? How can we improve motivation to en-joy each other's company? How can these interactions be infused throughout the toddler's waking hours?

This approach involves "social" goals for both interaction partners. We work with the family to increase the toddler's social responsiveness to contingencies arranged by the parent. For parents, we teach a basic interaction approach that the research literature suggests will increase overall responsiveness between the parent and child. (This approach includes attending to contextual variables, arranging the environment, setting the occasion for and responding to the child's social attempts and approximations, and responding in a way that is social and fun.) To help parents remember the components of a basic teaching interaction, we chose the acronym DANCE. This acronym was also developed to highlight Hart and Risley's (1999) metaphor regarding the "social dance" between parents and toddlers and to hopefully help parents understand the responsive and coordinated nature of the teaching interactions with their toddlers. Each component of the acronym will be described in detail later.

Because the children in our project are so young and the social interactions between any parent and toddler are less complex than with older children, the topography, or *what* we teach the parents to increase quality social interactions, is a relatively simple response. This is sufficient as long as we can achieve a point where the parent and child maintain and prolong the interactions with one another without our support.

The parents learn to target at least two toddler behaviors that the literature suggests will increase overall social opportunities—1) social attending, and 2) play. These are child behaviors that are more likely to produce generative and pervasive changes over time (Rosales-Ruiz & Baer, 1997). The first, social attending, involves the toddler orienting (eye gaze, body movements) to the parent. Previous research has shown that parents have learned to increase social gaze in toddlers with autism and that this appears to produce larger gains such as joint attention and increased social interactions. This teaching target is also supported by more basic research. For example, toddler research data suggest that behaviors such as the *lack* of differential eye gaze towards parents may be related to arrested developmental trajectories of social behavior (Jones and Klin, 2008).

The second target we teach is play. Play is considered central to a child's development, and children with autism have difficulties related to play and diversity of interests (American Psychiatric Association, 2000). Play is especially important for children with autism; it allows increasingly complex and enjoyable contact with diverse activities and social opportunities. It is generally agreed that to be considered play, it must be an activity that the child enjoys and that is chosen, not instructed or forced. For that reason, we are interested in helping parents increase the number of events that are playful and social. We do this in several ways. We introduce the parent to the concept of preference assessments, and interest expansion (Alai-Rosales, Zeug & Baynham, 2008), and we model and brainstorm ideas for new ways to playfully interact given each toddler's preferences. Furthermore, with this playful and social approach, parents learn to use consequences in ways that the research suggests produce favorable social outcomes for children and to choose activities that may increase affectionate responses. Frequently, the play responses are as simple as tickle games, airplane rides, puppets making funny noises, squirting water guns, playing chase, and dumping items with exaggerated facial expressions and sound effects.

Not surprisingly, the kinds of behaviors that parents of toddlers are often most concerned about are the toddler goals described above and that are supported in the literature. For this reason, our primary focus in the Sunny Starts program is teaching parents to increase the contexts for social attending and enjoyable social play interactions.

Working Assumptions

Sunny Starts is a behavioral intervention program, not a model. Although the basic goals have remained the same since the program's inception in 2003, the specific procedures have evolved in response to new research evidence and feedback from participants. We have three basic assumptions underlying our work.

Our first assumption is that our program will change as new data are available and as families tell us what they find most useful, effective, and life enhancing. There are several sources of research evidence we turn to when trying to improve our practice: interventions in autism (e.g., National Standards Project, 2009); infant-toddler research in autism (e.g., Green, Brennan, & Fein, 2002; Stahmer, & Ingersoll, 2004); parent support and training (e.g., Dunst & Kassow, 2004); child development (e.g., National Scientific Council on the Developing Child, 2004); and social behavior as it relates to parent-child relationships (e.g., Dunst, 2004) and adult learning (e.g., Trivette, Dunst, Hamby, & O'Herin, 2009). Finally, we refer to a growing body of research aimed specifically at parents and their toddlers with autism (Brookman-Frazee, 2004; Kasari, Gulsrud, Wong, Kwon, & Locke, 2010; Landa, Holman, O'Neill, & Stuart, 2010; Schertz and Odom, 2007; Vismara & Rogers, 2008; Vismara, Colombi, & Rogers, 2009).

When implementing practices from these sources, we work within the framework of applied behavior analysis; that is, we take a natural science approach to understanding and trying to improve family life. We assume that there are lawful patterns of behavior and that scientific method (behavioral descriptions, direct observations, and controlled introduction of teaching conditions) and social validation can help us identify and manage those patterns to the benefit of children and families (Baer, Wolf, & Risley, 1968). To that end, we collect data on parent and child progress and we rely on that data to inform program changes. We also value the opinions and feedback from the families we serve. Table 1 provides an example of our current satisfaction and feedback survey. To summarize, we keep abreast of research developments and we ensure that our families make progress and that they value the process and the outcomes. If research, individual family data, or parent feedback suggests a better course of action, we change.

Our second assumption is that parents have a special role as full collaborators during their children's early years. Our goal is that all families should be treated with kindness, dignity, respect, and sensitivity to their particular family culture and values. Along these lines, we try to acknowledge that all parents bring expertise and strengths to the intervention efforts and that they have the right and the responsibility for making choices and having control at every point in the program. This approach is supported by research on parent intervention partnerships.

Furthermore, full family participation and consideration is in keeping with our notions of social behavior; anything we teach occurs within the context of the family's ecology. Our goal is to help support events that will increase the overall health of the family ecosystem. In our case, this translates to direct teaching of parent and child social responses as well as careful attention to setting factors that may affect the ecosystem (e.g., family supports and resources, time management and scheduling, home safety and environmental arrangements, well-being of siblings, grandparent attitudes and interactions, etc.). We work with families to achieve an "ecological fit" with what they are learning and teaching. This is in keeping with the view that each member of the family affects one another and that a parent training intervention should be integrated into daily family life for everyone's betterment (Lutzker & Campbell, 1994).

Finally, we assume Sunny Starts is the first of many intervention steps for the family over the course of their child's life. This program is intended to be a prelude and a complement to an Early and Intensive Behavioral Intervention (EIBI), not a replacement. While our data indicate that the program has produced positive quantifiable outcomes, a larger body of research indicates that children with ASDs will require longer, intensive, and sustained interventions to increase overall functioning over the course of their lifetimes (Johnson & Meyers, 2007; Matson & Smith, 2010) and that families will continue to require support as they navigate services over time (Mayville & Letso, 2010). Sunny Starts is just a beginning point.

Table 1. Parent Feedback Survey Example

Please rate your satisfaction:	not satisfied	very satisfied	Please answer these questions as honestly as possible to help improve our program.
Overall Satisfaction			
My child learned meaningful skills.	0 1 2 3 4 5 6 7		What brought you to Sunny Starts?
I learned skills to help my child.	0 1 2 3 4 5 6 7		What did you do during training sessions?
Sunny Starts helped our family.	0 1 2 3 4 5 6 7		
Satisfaction with Program			
Components	0 1 2 3 4 5 6 7		What did you learn?
Professional staff	0 1 2 3 4 5 6 7		
Clinical facilities	0 1 2 3 4 5 6 7		What did your child learn?
Intake process	0 1 2 3 4 5 6 7		
Community networking resources	0 1 2 3 4 5 6 7		What did you like best about training?
Assessment procedures	0 1 2 3 4 5 6 7		
Goal setting process	0 1 2 3 4 5 6 7		What did you like least about training?
Parent training techniques	0 1 2 3 4 5 6 7		
Home support and assistance	0 1 2 3 4 5 6 7		What would you change?
Exit report and transition	0 1 2 3 4 5 6 7		
Additional comments:			Is Sunny Starts a useful program and, if so, why?

Service Sequence

Overview: Table 2 provides an overview of the Sunny Starts service sequence. Families attend a one-hour session either once or twice per week for a period of five to ten weeks. The schedule depends on the family's logistical requirements (work, distance to drive, nap schedules, other appointments), although most sessions run in the mornings. A lead coach (the first author, a professor, or a senior graduate student) and a coach in training (a junior graduate student) conduct the sessions. The skills required of a lead coach include:

- Friendly parent interactions skills (hopeful, attentive, kind)
- Excellent communication skills (responsive, clear, accurate)
- Master autism interventions skills (BACB Autism Task List)
- Master toddler play skill repertoire (fun, interactive, responsive)
- Advanced training skills (narrating, instructing, modeling, feedback)
- Organization and technical skills (data, schedules, materials)

The staff engage in a series of activities with the family: An initial assessment and relationship-building phase, periodic assessments in the home and clinic, an intensive training period, and a transition and exit phase. Each of these activities will be described in detail.

Table 2.   Timeline of Services

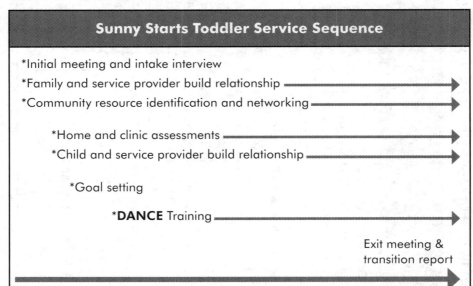

Sunny Starts Toddler Service Sequence
*Initial meeting and intake interview
*Family and service provider build relationship ⟶
*Community resource identification and networking ⟶
*Home and clinic assessments ⟶
*Child and service provider build relationship ⟶
*Goal setting
***DANCE** Training ⟶
Exit meeting & transition report

Intake Meeting and Interviews: During the initial meeting, we describe the program, review a service agreement that outlines expectations for staff and parents, and answer questions. Before any formal training begins, we want to do our best to provide information about Sunny Starts so that parents, along with other family members, can decide if this is the right time and program for their family. If the family chooses to continue with Sunny Starts, we start the interview process, which includes an assessment packet. Usually, parents prefer to fill the information out at home and then we ask clarification and follow-up questions in our next meeting. The questions address: 1) family goals and history; 2) social-communication skills and contexts of use; 3) play and imitation skills and contexts of engagement; 4) preferences, with a special emphasis on play activities and social events; and 5) child and family daily and weekly schedule.

The interview is five pages and the completion and follow-up process can take between thirty minutes and several hours, depending on how much the parent would like to talk. The interview and follow-up not only provides information that informs training, but also serves as the beginning of the relationship-building process between the Sunny Starts staff and the family.

Relationship Building: This starts at the beginning of the program and continues throughout the training process. It includes rapport with the parent (Ingersoll & Dvortcsak, 2006) and with the child (Carr et al., 1994). This is one of the most important parts of the program. With the parents, we spend time telling about ourselves and learning about them—as parents and as individuals. With the children, we spend time playing and sampling different toys and games. These activities help us get to know the family and help them get to know us: We try to learn ways to communicate effectively, learn what members of the family like and dislike, and learn what parts of family life are difficult and what parts are easy. All of this helps inform the training and reminds us that we share a common goal: to help the family.

It is also during relationship building activities that we discover additional support needs. For example, the family might need counseling, financial assistance, or additional therapeutic care. In these cases, we make referrals and help the family seek the additional supports needed.

Community Networking: Often Sunny Starts is one of the first points of intervention contact for the family. Typically the child has just received a diagnosis (or concerns have been formally addressed but no diagnostic label assigned) and family members are beginning to navigate institutional systems and figure out what they need to do to help their child. As we are building rapport and conducting assessments, we are also providing materials (a community resource book, websites, books, articles, DVDs), making contacts and introductions to other agencies, and answering many, many questions. This continues throughout the process. Parents have reported this to be an

Sunny Starts Data Sheet

Session Date:_____ Scoring Date:_____ Observer:_____ Ob1 Ob2

Child:_____ Parent:_____ Condition:_____

Count Home helper sheets completed since last session?   Y N

#	Event	Parent		Child			Parent	
		Decide High Pref	Arrange	Attending	Verbal	Play Action	Now	
1			Enviro Model				Expand	Social Tangible
2			Enviro Model				Expand	Social Tangible
3			Enviro Model				Expand	Social Tangible
4			Enviro Model				Expand	Social Tangible
5			Enviro Model				Expand	Social Tangible
6			Enviro Model				Expand	Social Tangible
7			Enviro Model				Expand	Social Tangible
8			Enviro Model				Expand	Social Tangible
9			Enviro Model				Expand	Social Tangible
10			Enviro Model				Expand	Social Tangible
11			Enviro Model				Expand	Social Tangible
12			Enviro Model				Expand	Social Tangible
13			Enviro Model				Expand	Social Tangible
14			Enviro Model				Expand	Social Tangible
15			Enviro Model				Expand	Social Tangible
16			Enviro Model				Expand	Social Tangible
17			Enviro Model				Expand	Social Tangible
18			Enviro Model				Expand	Social Tangible
19			Enviro Model				Expand	Social Tangible
20			Enviro Model				Expand	Social Tangible
21			Enviro Model				Expand	Social Tangible
22			Enviro Model				Expand	Social Tangible
Total								
Total Teaching Episodes								

Enjoy rating for this session:

Parent Interest: 0) Not interested 1) Somewhat interested 2) Mostly interested 3) Enthusiastically interested

Child Interest: 0) Not interested 1) Somewhat interested 2) Mostly interested 3) Enthusiastically interested

Parent Affect: 0) Unhappy 1) Nervous, Anxious 2) Calm 3) Happy, exuberant

Child Affect: 0) Unhappy 1) Nervous, Anxious 2) Calm 3) Happy, exuberant

Figure 1. Example of Session Data Sheet

important part of the program, and the networking has been what typically results in the child's next or concurrent intervention opportunity.

Home and Clinic Assessments and Data Collection: We assess the effects of our training efforts in two ways: through direct observations and through interviews and surveys. All direct measures are adapted from behavioral definitions found in the intervention literature, and from interview protocols and ratings used with families and further developed within thesis projects as part of our graduate training program.

To objectively evaluate session progress, we collect video samples and make direct observations of the behaviors we would like to increase. Five-minute samples of parent-child interactions are collected at home and in the clinic. Clinic samples are collected at the very beginning of every clinic session, allowing us to see what is going well and what we should work on during the training session. Home samples are taken to see whether the DANCE training effects have generalized to the home. In both cases, we count what happens during the five-minute sample. An example of our current data sheet is displayed in Figure 1 on the previous page.

At this point in time, we count the events (play activities and games), parent teaching episodes (use of high preference events, environmental arrangements, responsive models, language expansions, social and tangible consequences), and child skills (attending, verbal, play actions). These measures allow us to see whether the parent and child are making progress. Overall session ratings are made of child and parent interest and affect. This helps us monitor overall enjoyment and comfort with the training process. For research purposes, we are also going back and counting the way children are directing social attention between parents and activities. This is called "coordinated joint attention" and appears to be important to later social development (Brunisma & Keogel, 2004).

Goal Setting: After the third session, the coaches and the parents review the assessment information and look at graphed baseline data (parent DANCE components and child attending and play responses) from the first series of assessments (usually three from the clinic and one from home). At that point, we also examine basic skill areas thought to be important for toddlers with autism (Table 3, page 36) and talk about how social attending and social play fit within the "big picture." The overview we created was informed by autism intervention books (e.g., Lovaas, 2003; McEachin & Leaf, 1999) and by infant and toddler parenting books (e.g., Brazelton, 2006; Sears et al., 2003) and was designed to help parents see the overall goals and the possible component skills needed to reach the goal areas. Upon reviewing all the information, the parents and coaches determine the specifics of how attending and play will be addressed and whether additional communication skills should also be considered.

Table 3. Planning Guide for Toddler Skills

Overarching Goal			
To increase responsiveness, enjoyment and benefit from the social environment; to learn from others and develop loving family relationships and close friendships over the course of a lifetime.			
Domain	**Early Social**	**Early Interests and Activities**	**Early Communication**
Master Goals	enjoys communicating and sharing activities with others; develops attachments to widening circle of people	enjoys playing with a wide range of activities alone and with others	communicates own likes, dislikes, and interests; responds to communications of others
Skills	social attending, affectionate gestures, turn taking, motor, object imitation, and vocal imitation	sampling, selecting, and manipulating play and daily life objects within and across classes	functional (varied forms) for expressive and receptive communication

DANCE Training: Training begins after initial assessments are completed, rapport is developed with both the child and the parent, and goals are specified. A mnemonic, DANCE, is used to help parents remember each of the teaching components and to emphasize the interactive and enjoyable purpose. DANCE stands for:

- **D**ecide,
- **A**rrange,
- **N**ow,
- **C**ount, and
- **E**njoy.

Each of these words describes a collection of procedures represented in a teaching interaction. These procedures are similar to and/or derived from several sources describing naturalistic teaching interaction procedures for preschoolers and toddlers with disabilities and from the naturalistic parent training research described earlier.

The Teaching DANCE involves five parts:

> **1.** _Decide._ Parents are taught to decide upon favorable teaching times for themselves and their children (e.g., the parent has

few competing responsibilities, the child is rested, diapers are clean, the parent has chosen a skill/response to teach).

2. *Arrange.* Parents are taught to arrange the environment in order to maximize learning opportunities (e.g., evaluate their child's preferences, ensure the availability of a variety of high preference items, have methods to regulate and rotate access to the items, ensure that all materials are safe and working properly).

3. *Now!* Parents are taught to respond effectively to their child's approximations. This includes responding immediately and with enthusiastic affect when their child approximates to the desired goal responses; adjusting subsequent opportunities based on their child's response; and working in short, successful episodes that include fun play (from the child's point of view), taking turns within activities, and rotating activities.

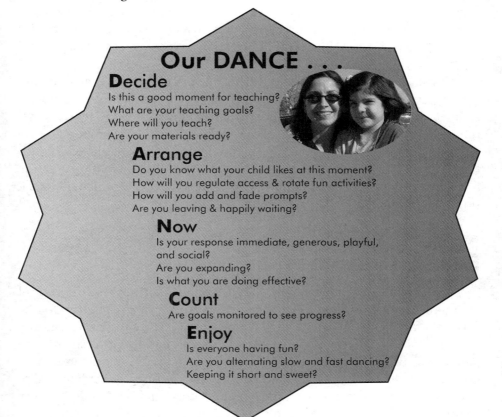

Our DANCE . . .

Decide
Is this a good moment for teaching?
What are your teaching goals?
Where will you teach?
Are your materials ready?

Arrange
Do you know what your child likes at this moment?
How will you regulate access & rotate fun activities?
How will you add and fade prompts?
Are you leaving & happily waiting?

Now
Is your response immediate, generous, playful, and social?
Are you expanding?
Is what you are doing effective?

Count
Are goals monitored to see progress?

Enjoy
Is everyone having fun?
Are you alternating slow and fast dancing?
Keeping it short and sweet?

Figure 2. DANCE Management Reminder

4. *Count.* Parents learn to count occurrences of goal responses at home.

5. *Enjoy.* Parents are encouraged to adjust their teaching in ways that make both the child and the parent happy and comfortable during teaching interactions.

In the first training session, the coach describes the teaching procedures to the parent, models for the parent, and practices with the parent. The coach and parents then discuss changes and retry the procedures. Parents are given a short manual describing the procedures and a refrigerator magnet summarizing the procedures. The magnet is personalized and has a picture of the child and parent(s) embedded along with the DANCE components. An example is shown in Figure 2 on the previous page.

At the end of each training session, the parent and coach review the session and determine family goals for the week. It is important for the coach and parent to understand how the "DANCE" best fits into the family's natural ecology, so several variables are considered, including the family's current routines, activities, and schedule. Taken together, the parent and coach determine the date, time, and conditions under which the parent will practice and implement the "DANCE." This information is written on the "Home Helper," which is displayed in Figure 3.

It usually takes two or three sessions to work out the right amount and type of activity that will be done at home—*all* team members over- or underestimate what can be done and under what conditions. Furthermore, sometimes scheduling time to have teaching interactions is challenging and we will spend additional efforts in helping the family increase relaxed interaction time and/or gain more social support at home. In combination with the home assessments, this is our effort to promote a context in which the social skills and interactions will generalize and sustain.

Family Outcomes

We would like to end our description of Sunny Starts by sharing some of our families' stories and data. Figure 4 presents an overview of progress for the first eight families that went through our program. The data are collapsed and averaged for ease of presentation. Generally, during baseline assessments, the parents had a very limited number of teaching interactions (most parents had none and a few had one every five minutes). Before training, the children were not attending to their parents, not communicating, and not playing in very complex or safe ways. There was also very little coordinated attention. (Most children exhibited no attention and two children had very low rates.)

Sunny Starts Home Helper

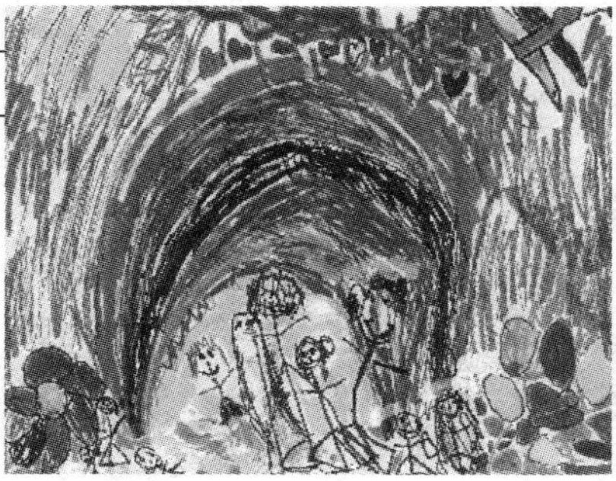

Date:_____ Parent:_____

Child:_____

Progress ⬆ ⬇ ➡

Training Session Goal:

DANCE Practice Reminders:

Decide

Arrange

Now!

Count

Enjoy!

Home Planning:

Practice time(s):_____ Place(s):_____

Count:_____

Activity Highlight—*What were your most enjoyable play activities?*

Next Tele Training Session:_____ Next Clinic Training Session:_____

Be sure to write questions on the back!

Figure 3. Ecological Integration

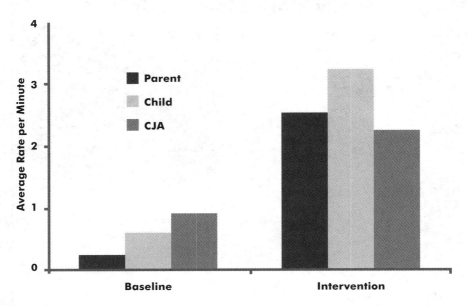

Sunny Start Outcomes: First Eight Families

Figure 4. Parent Teacher Episodes, Child Responding, and Coordinated Joint Attention Across Assessment Conditions

Following DANCE training, on average, parents were providing 6 teaching opportunities per minute and child goal responses were in tandem with the parents'. Furthermore, the children were spending much of the time in coordinated attention with the parents, an average of ten episodes per minute. In effect, what we see is that the parents and toddlers increase the number of responsive events to one another. This is social progress, and, in each case, parents have expressed their happiness at the changes and improvements. Here are a few of their stories:

The Mancini Family

Danny, a contented toddler with big dark brown eyes, arrived with his own entourage! His mother, sisters, cousins, and grandparents all came to the first session. Each and every family member was smiling and eager to learn. Olivia Mancini, his mother, received most of the direct training. But his father and other family members also participated and contributed to the effort.

At the time he began in Sunny Starts, Danny had already been attending a private early intervention program. In this program, Danny had learned to point to get access to items that he wanted (for example, his pacifier or chips) and Olivia had learned how to require him to point before she gave him something. She was very good at this and very proud that he had learned to gesture with meaning. His pointing, however, appeared to be very "unsocial." That is, he pointed to get access to an item and then went away to his own isolated activity. Not only did he not make eye contact, but he actively appeared to avoid looking at anyone. So, following a period of rapport building, we started to work with Olivia on transferring what she had learned to do with the pointing to Danny's social attending and to develop social games that he would like and that would maintain his attention.

Olivia learned to apply the DANCE components very quickly and only two areas required more extensive brainstorming—feedback and revision— the timing of event delivery and developing activities that were social and preferred. We worked on the timing (immediate is better so that the child understands that eye contact produces fun) by taking turns practicing and helping each other immediately catch the social gaze (or an approximation to it). The first thing we discovered was that (like many of the toddlers) Danny loved "tickle monster" games. This was easy to incorporate into a requirement to look and to do immediately. We would creep our fingers up his legs with an expectant look, saying, "Here comes the tickle monster. . ." and when Danny looked, we would say "Arghhh!!!!" and tickle him. He loved this activity and would pull our arms up, raise his eyebrows, and look expectantly. This activity we could further develop using songs and other phrases.

Along the same lines, to expand play activities, we experimented with the toys at Danny's home and in our clinic. We tried both conventional and nonconventional uses. For example, we used the plastic balls to one game to make another game with a bucket. We would take turns throwing balls into the buckets and then dump them on Danny's head. This produced delightful giggles and lots of social eye gaze. For each ball that was thrown, and for the big finale (the bucket on his head), he was required to look. The wonderful thing was that Danny kept laughing and looking at his mom and all of us even after the balls were delivered and the bucket was dumped!

Several months after Sunny Starts had ended, his family sent us a video of Olivia successfully teaching Danny to say "Mama." At the end of the video clip they are both smiling at the camera.

The Ameen Family

Our nickname for Shirin was "Angel." She had long golden curls, was very quiet, loved to cuddle and be close to adults, and always had to have one hand touching her mother. She did not make eye contact, talk, or play in any conventional sense. She had several objects that she liked to carry around and would become upset if they were removed. She also was deeply inter-ested in price tag stickers.

Shirin's family had recently immigrated, both parents were highly edu-cated, and she had several older brothers. At the time of the intake interview, they reported being isolated from friends and family and expressed shock and sadness about the diagnosis of autism. As the sessions progressed, it be-came clear that the family was in crisis. We continued rapport building, com-munity networking, and helping the Ameens to access Early and Intensive Behavioral Intervention and sibling support programs. We attempted to start DANCE training, but the family was very concerned with the other matters and asked to stop participation.

Several months later, the Ameen family reported that conditions had improved. One of the grandmothers had moved in, the siblings were receiv-ing training and support, and Shirin was enrolled in an intervention program for 20 hours per week. The intervention program was teaching Shirin new skills and also allowed some respite for Zainab, her mother. Upon the family's request, we reinstituted DANCE training. The initial assessments still showed no social attending and very little play. Once training began, Zainab quickly learned the DANCE techniques. Shirin continued to sit in her mother's lap at times but also began to sit across from her to play the games and activities we introduced. Her eye contact increased dramatically and we were able to expand her interest in price tag stickers to play scenes and to book stickers that we could do together. We also introduced play food items that were simi-lar to the objects she carried around. Zainab would "eat" the play food (with very silly facial expressions) that Shirin handed her. This produced beautiful social attending and deep giggles from mother and daughter!

The Zang Family

Our first comment after meeting Roger Zang and his 18-month-old twins was "Wow!" The twins were adorable, freckled toddlers with abun-dant energy. Within minutes after they entered the clinic, they had explored and dumped every accessible item. Like Shirin, they did not talk or babble, had very limited conventional play activity, and made no eye contact. In this case, the twins' father, Roger, was the primary person to be trained. Both parents worked, but Roger's schedule allowed more flexibility to attend the Sunny Starts sessions. He would tape each session and then he and his wife, Emily, would watch the DANCE training session and practice on their own. Each week, they would come in with a list of ideas and questions written on the back of the "Home Helper" sheets. They were very active collaborators throughout the entire program.

The Zangs had two sets of twins with autism spectrum disorders. The older twins were described by the parents as having Asperger syndrome. The younger twins had a diagnosis of PDD-NOS. Both Emily and Roger were quite good at teaching and interacting with the older boys. They found, however, that it was more of a challenge to identify interests and "focus" the younger boys. Our clinic sessions were devoted to finding ways to regulate access to high preference events (containers they couldn't open worked well) and to developing social games that involved a lot of roughhousing and movement (for example, pillow tosses, jumping on trampolines together). It was also very important to help create an evening routine schedule that allowed the parents to implement the DANCE procedures with each of their younger sons and still interact with the older boys. Eventually, the older siblings began to help the parents with the teaching interactions in the evenings. Everyone was dancing!

Conclusion

To watch us dance is to hear our hearts speak.
~Hopi Indian Saying

Sunny Starts is a short-term parent training program designed to help parents teach and respond to the social and play behavior of their children. It is modeled after several naturalistic programs for children with autism. Each family has been unique in terms of implementing the Sunny Starts DANCE procedures. Some families faced difficulties with specific procedures, some with larger life circumstances, and some with logistical arrangements. In all cases, the families have reported satisfaction with services and have observed meaningful changes. Sunny Starts is designed to lift the hearts of families and to be a starting point for increasing skilled social dancing between parents and their toddlers with ASD.

References

Ala'i-Rosales, S., Zeug, N. M., & Baynam, T. (2008). The development of interests in children with autism: A method to establish baselines for analyses and evaluation. *Behavioral Development Bulletin, 14,* 3-16.

American Psychiatric Association (2000). *Diagnostic and statistical manual of mental disorders IV.* Washington, DC: American Psychiatric Association.

Baer, D. M., Wolf, M. M., & Risley, T. R. (1968). Some current dimensions of applied behavior analysis. *Journal of Applied Behavior Analysis, 1,* 91-97.

Brazelton, T. B., & Sparrow, J. D. (2006). *Touchpoints.* Cambridge, MA: Da Capo Press

Brookman-Frazee, L. (2004). Using parent/clinician partnerships in parent education programs for children with autism. *Journal of Positive Behavior Interventions, 6,* 195–213.

Bruinsma, Y., Koegel, R.L., & Koegel, L.K. (2004). Joint attention and children with autism: A review of the literature. *Mental Retardation and Developmental Disabilities,* 10, 169-175.

Carr, E. G., Levin, L., McConnachie, G., Carlson, J. E., Kemp, D. C., & Smith, C. E. (1994). *Communication-based intervention for problem behavior.* Baltimore: Paul H. Brookes.

Dunst, C. J., & Kassow, D. Z. (2004). Characteristics of interventions promoting parental sensitivity to child behavior. *Bridges, 2,* 1-17.

Green, G., Brennan, L. C., & Fein, D. (2002). Intensive behavioral treatment for a toddler at high risk for autism. *Behavior Modification, 26,* 69-102.

Haring, T. G. (1992). The context of social competence: Relations, relationships, and generalization (Chapter 12). In Odom, S.L., McConnell, S.R., & McEvoy, M.A. (Eds.), *Social competence of young children with disabilities: Issues and strategies for intervention.* Baltimore, MD: Paul H. Brookes.

Hart, B., & Risley, T. R. (1995). *Meaningful differences in the everyday experience of young American children.* Baltimore: Paul H. Brookes.

Hart, B., & Risley, T. R. (1999). *The social world of children: Learning to talk.* Baltimore: Paul H. Brookes.

Hartman, D. (1999, Fall). The engaged university: Thinking about the new millennium. *Sustainable Community Review,* 12-17.

Ingersoll, B., & Dvortcsak, A. (2006). Including parent training in the early childhood special education curriculum for children with autism spectrum disorders. *Journal of Positive Behavior Interventions, 8,* 79-87.

Johnson, C. P., & Myers, S. M. (2007). Identification and evaluation of children with autism spectrum disorder. *Pediatrics, 120,* 1183-1215.

Kasari, C., Gulsrud, A. C., Wong, C., Kwon, S., & Locke, J. (2010). Randomized controlled caregiver mediated joint engagement intervention for toddlers with autism. *Journal of Autism and Developmental Disorders, 40,* 1045-1056.

Klin, A., & Jones, W. (2008). Altered face scanning and impaired recognition of biological motion in a 15-month-old infant with autism. *Developmental Science, 11,* 40-46.

Landa, R., Holman, K., O'Neill, A., & Stuart, E. (2011). Intervention targeting development of socially synchronous engagement in toddlers with autism spectrum disorder: A randomized controlled trial. *Journal of Child Psychology and Psychiatry,* 52, 13-21.

Leaf, R., & McEachin, J. (1999). *A work in progress.* New York, NY: DRL Books.

Lovaas, O. I. (2003). *Teaching individuals with developmental delays.* Austin, TX: Pro-Ed.

Lutzker, J. R., & Cambell, R. (1994). *Ecobehavioral family interventions in developmental disorders.* Pacific Grove, CA: Brooks/Cole Publishing.

Marcus, L. M., Kunce, L. J., & Schopler, E. (2005). Working with families. In: Volkmar, F., Paul, R., Klin, A., & Cohen, D. (Eds.), *Handbook of autism and pervasive developmental disorders (Vol. 2): Assessment, interventions, and policy* (3rd ed.). Hoboken, NJ: Wiley.

Matson, J. L., & Smith, K. R. M. (2008). Current status of intensive behavioral interventions for young children with autism and PDDNOS. *Research in Autism Spectrum Disorders, 2,* 60-74.

Mayville, E. A., & Letso, S. (2010). Family and community curricular content for training in applied behavior analysis and autism. *European Journal of Behavior Analysis, 12,* 229-238.

McConnell, S. (2002). Interventions to facilitate social interaction for young children with autism: Review of available research and recommendations for educational intervention and future research. *Journal of Autism and Developmental Disorders, 32,* 351-372.

Miller, S. (1994). Peer coaching within an early childhood interdisciplinary setting. *Intervention in School and Clinic, 30,* 109-113.

National Scientific Council on the Developing Child. (2004/9). *Young children develop in an environment of relationships.* Working Paper No. 1. Retrieved from www. developingchild.net.

Noonan, M., & McCormick, L. (2006). Young children with disabilities in natural environments: Methods and procedures. Baltimore, MD: Paul H. Brookes.

Odom, S., McConnell, S., & McEvoy, M. (Eds.). *Social competence of young children with disabilities: Issues and strategies for intervention.* Baltimore, MD: Paul H. Brookes.

Rosales-Ruiz, J., & Baer, D. M. (1997). Behavioral cusps: A developmental and pragmatic construct for behavior analysis. *Journal of Applied Behavior Analysis, 30,* 533-544.

Schertz, H. H., & Odom, S. L. (2007). Promoting joint attention in toddlers with autism: A parent-mediated developmental model. *Journal of Autism and Developmental Disabilities, 37,* 1562-1575.

Sears, W., Sears, M., Sears, R., & Sears, J. (2003). *The baby book: Everything you need to know about your baby from birth to age two* (Rev. ed.). New York, NY: Little, Brown, & Co.

Skinner, B. F. (1953). *Science and human behavior.* New York, NY: Macmillan Publishers.

Stahmer, A. C., & Ingersoll, B. (2004). Inclusive programming for toddlers with autism spectrum disorders: Outcomes from the children's toddler school. *Journal of Positive Behavior Interventions, 6,* 67-82.

Symon, J. B. (2005). Expanding interventions for children with autism: Parents as trainers. *Journal of Positive Behavior Interventions, 7,* 159-173.

Trivette, C. M., Dunst, C. J., Hamby, D. W., & O'Herin, C. E. (2009). Characteristics and consequences of adult learning methods and strategies. *Practical Evaluation Reports, 2*(1), 1–32.

Vismara, L.A., Colombi, C., & Rogers, S.J. (2009). Can one hour per week of therapy lead to lasting changes in young children with autism? *Autism, 13,* 93-115.

Vismara, L. A., & Rogers, S. J. (2008). The early start Denver model: A case study of innovative practice. *Journal of Early Intervention, 31,* 91-108.

Wolfberg, P. J. (2003). *Peer play and the autism spectrum: The art of guiding children's socialization and imagination.* Shawnee Mission, KS: Autism Asperger Publishing Company.

Author's Note:

Thank you to all the students who assisted with the development of Sunny Starts: Katherine Laino, Amanda Besner, Elizabeth Goettl, Andrea Newcomer, Jessica Broome, Robin Kuhn, Donna Dempsey, Lashanna Brunson, Megan Geving, Allison Jones, Nicole Suchomel, Nicole Zeug, Sarah Ewing, Barbie Carlson, Mona Alhaddad, Larisa Maxwell, Heather Barahona, Julie Winn Greer, Kellyn Johnson, and Victoria White.

3

An Evidence-Based Social Skills Group for Children with Autism

Marjorie H. Charlop and Melaura Andree Erickson

Social skills are a set of behaviors that consist of the ability to relate to others in a reciprocally reinforcing manner, and the ability to adapt social behaviors to different contexts (Schopler & Mesibov, 1986). Children with autism display profound deficits in social behavior (Kanner, 1943; Rimland, 1964; Rutter, 1978), and one of the defining characteristics of this disorder is an unwillingness to engage in social interactions (American Psychiatric Association, 2000).

Social deficits are evident from an extremely early age in individuals with autism and persist throughout development. As infants, they may not reach out in anticipation of being picked up or may not mold to their parents' bodies when held (Charlop-Christy, Schreibman, Pierce, & Kurtz, 1998). They may also display less obvious patterns of attachment to their parents and may demonstrate little to no separation distress that is common in typically developing children (Weiss & Harris, 2001a). For example, infants with autism may cry when their parents approach and may seem quite content to be alone in their cribs. An additional deficit that first appears during infancy in individuals with autism is lack of eye contact and gaze aversion (American Psychiatric Association, 1994). Affectionate gestures such as hugs and kisses may also not be sought or given.

As children with autism get older, these social deficits continue and other deficiencies in social behavior also become apparent. Young preschool-age children with autism have difficulties with joint attention, imitation, and responding to social stimuli. For example, young children generally like to imitate things that adults do, such as using tools like their dad or cooking like their mom. This kind of imitation occurs spontaneously in typically developing children, while children with autism often have to be taught simple imitations such as clapping hands or standing up. This lack of ability or interest in imitating others interferes with development of a variety of social skills learned through imitation of adults or peers.

An additional area of impairment seen in young children with autism that interferes with early socialization is an atypical and delayed progression of play skills. While children with autism may engage in solitary play, they show little, if any, interest in initiating playful interactions with other children. Further, the solitary play exhibited by young children with autism often lacks creativity and is rather characterized by the use of a limited number of preferred toys and behavior that is stereotypic or repetitive (e.g., staring at the wheels of a car as they turn, lining up toy cars). In children with autism who do develop some imaginary play, the scenarios are often simple and repetitive and lack the variation that is common in same age typically developing peers.

As children with autism enter the school-age years, social deficits become even more apparent at a time when socialization is of extreme importance. School-age children with autism often fail to initiate or respond to interactions with peers. When they do initiate interactions, it is often in an atypical or inappropriate way (e.g., excessive touching to gain attention or being too close to the peer). An additional deficit that hinders social relationships at this age is an inability to initiate or sustain conversations. Approximately 50 percent of children with autism fail to acquire functional speech (Charlop & Haymes, 1994; Rimland, 1964; Rutter, 1978).

Children with autism who do acquire expressive language often demonstrate speech that is limited to simple responses to questions, or to brief expressions of a need or desire (e.g., "I want cookie") (Schreibman, 1988). This type of speech differs from conversational speech. Conversational speech requires the use of multiple, complex language skills including initiation and expansion of a conversational topic, establishing an interactive "to and fro" pattern of a conversation, and maintaining a verbal exchange (Charlop & Milstein, 1989; Charlop-Christy & Kelso, 2003). There are important consequences that result from children with autism failing to develop this type of conversational speech. For example, it eliminates opportunities to have extended verbal interactions with others and to learn through social interaction. Therefore, this deficit exacerbates the severe social withdrawal and aloofness already common in many children with autism and may have significant impacts on their future development and life.

Inadequate social skills characteristic in children with autism hinder development by:

1. increasing behavior problems that result from not having the appropriate skills for social interactions,
2. increasing the likelihood for maladaptive behavior later in life, and
3. decreasing the positive developmental support and learning opportunities found in successful peer relationships.

Further, children with social skill delays are unpopular, not accepted by their peers, and are frequently subject to negative stereotypes. However, research has shown that social interest and social skills development are among the most crucial variables determining long-term adjustment and prognosis for individuals with autism (Matson & Swiezy, 1994). Children with autism who learn to seek out and enjoy social interactions with others and understand appropriate social "rules" have much better prognoses and chances for living and functioning independently. Therefore, there is a need to develop interventions that focus on teaching social skills to children so that they will become more successful in initiating and navigating social interactions. However, social skills interventions available for children with autism vary tremendously in their methodology and approach. One reason for this problem is the difficulty of defining social skills and the lack of a consistent definition across researchers and practitioners.

Defining "Social Skills"

The lack of a clear and consistent definition of social skills is seen in literature on neurotypical populations as well as populations with developmental disabilities such as autism. This absence of a clear definition has resulted in the prolonged development of assessment tools, confusion about what is being measured, and the use of vague terminology. It is often challenging to define social skills due to the wide variety of populations that have been studied (Matson & Swiezy, 1994). When discussed with regards to the general child population, the term "social skills" often focuses on sophisticated interpersonal skills, including relating, perspective taking, and empathy, whereas in populations with intellectual disabilities or other developmental delays, the same term encompasses a wider range of more rudimentary behaviors such as making eye contact and giving hugs.

While a variety of definitions of social skills have been proposed, common elements appear in the literature. Researchers often suggest that the concept of social skills includes perceptual, cognitive, and performance components (Bedell & Lennox, 1997. In studies with delayed populations, researchers often prefer a more limited definition of social skills, indicating that a simpler definition is more appropriate for lower functioning individuals who have extreme difficulty with complex cognitive behaviors such as perspective taking and interpersonal problem-solving. According to this perspective, individuals demonstrating appropriate social skills have the ability to adapt to their environment by exhibiting appropriate motor skills (e.g., hand waving, pointing, or giving hugs). Still another definition commonly used suggests that social skills include both cognitive and motor abilities. In such definitions, appropriate social skills would include the application of relevant motor, cognitive, and affective skills or behaviors according to the context. This definition will be adapted for the remainder of this chapter.

In addition to the difficulty of clearly defining social skills, it is also a challenge to distinguish between social skills and language/communication skills. While social and communicative skills are often studied separately, there has been a growing acknowledgement of their interrelatedness. Given that language is considered a primary mediator of social interaction and an inherent aspect of social development (Goldstein, Kaczmarek, Pennington, & Shafer, 1992), it is often difficult to consider the two skills independently. The relationship between the two skills becomes more evident when looking at how and when the two develop. The development of communication begins soon after birth within the context of social interaction with caregivers and eventually leads to the development of language (Prizant & Wetherby, 1990). As children grow older, they continue to enhance their communication skills, and this occurs within the context of social interactions. At the same time, children's communicative abilities assist them in becoming more socially competent. Throughout development, children continue to use language and communication to enhance their social interactions and use their social skills to enhance their language and communication. Therefore, it is difficult to study one of these areas of development without recognizing the other and the relationship between the two.

Despite the difficulty in determining a clear and consistent definition of social skills and in distinguishing social skills from communicative skills, there continues to be a need to develop effective interventions for social skill development. This need is especially important for children with autism, who do not develop social skills or demonstrate delays in social functioning. The National Autism Plan for Children recommended that children and adolescents with ASD should have access to planned, additional, individual and small group social skills opportunities tailored to their needs (National Initiative for Autism: Screening and Assessment [NIASA], 2003). Such treatment programs should consist of evidence-based interventions. One program that offers this type of social skills intervention is the Claremont Autism Center (CAC), discussed below.

The Claremont Autism Center's Social Skills Group Approach

The CAC is a treatment and research center for children with autism and their families. The center focuses on research addressing speech and language, motivation, and social skills. Behavioral intervention is applied via direct therapy with the children as well as parent training sessions. Children who are higher functioning and no longer require one-on-one therapy graduate into the center's social skills group. The social skills group offers a group approach that incorporates structured activities as well as less structured environments (e.g., recess) similar to those experienced by typically developing peers. A variety of procedures and intervention techniques (see Table 1 and descriptions on the next page) are used to develop and increase the use of appropriate social skill behaviors (see Table 2, page 53). While the procedures and social skills discussed are representative of what is targeted at the CAC, it is not an exhaustive list. Only procedures that have been empirically validated are implemented at the center and all social skills training sessions are videotaped and data are then taken.

While many intervention programs for children with ASD offer individualized treatment packages, the social skills group at the CAC focuses on teaching social skills in small group settings. There are several reasons why it is beneficial to target social skills during small group interventions as opposed to one-to-one instruction. First, opportunities for social interaction in the child's natural environment will most often occur in group settings. Further, generalization is more likely to occur when skills are taught in environments that closely resemble the environment to which the child will return (Stokes & Baer, 1977). Additionally, in group settings, children are able to practice learned social skills with a variety of peers. By training and practicing newly acquired skills with a number of exemplars (other children), generalization is more likely to occur. In addition to these benefits of using small group interventions to target social skills, Reichow & Volkmar (2010) found social skills groups to have met the highest level of evidence-based practice based on the criteria of evidence-based practice proposed by Reichow, Volkmar, & Cicchetti (2008).

The remainder of the chapter will describe how the center selects social skills to target in intervention, how we assess social skills, and the interventions used to train and maintain social competence.

Table 1. Interventions Used to Teach Social Skills

Procedure	Brief Description	Example of Social Skill Taught	Reference
Naturalistic Teaching Strategies (NaTS)	Teaching strategies that incorporate motivation, functional relationships, and facilitators of generalization	Pretend play	LaBelle (2002) Stahmer & Schreibman (1992)
Peer Mediated Strategies	Train neurotypical peers to initiate, prompt, and reinforce social interactions with children with autism	Joint attention and play	Zercher et al. (2001)
Video Modeling	Technique that involves demonstration of desired behaviors through video representation of the behavior	Sharing and social greetings	Simpson et al. (2004)
Scripts	Implementation of written or audio recorded scripts that provide models of the appropriate language to be learned	Joint attention behaviors	MacDuff et al. (2007)
Self-Management	Improve the social behavior of children with autism by teaching them to keep a count of the number of times they engage in the desired behavior or outcome	Eye contact and appropriate conversation	Koegel & Frea (1993)
Parent Training	Training parents to implement behavioral procedures to increase their child's use of social behaviors in the home and community	Initiations	Ingersoll & Gergans (2007)

Table 2. Operational Definitions of Social Skills Targets at the Claremont Autism Center

Social Skill	Operational Definition of Social Skill
Greetings	Child comes into contact with a peer for the first time or upon arriving at a new location, and says "hello" within 5 seconds. If the child is nonverbal, he or she will say hello by gesturing with hand within 5 seconds.
Eye Contact	Child must look directly at an adult or other child's eyes or in the near vicinity of the eyes for approximately 3 seconds.
Play	
Parallel Play	Children play adjacent to and within 4 feet (1.2 meters) of one another, but in a solitary manner. They are not interacting but playing near one another.
Cooperative Play	Children are within 1 foot (.33 m) of each other. Children may be playing with the same materials (e.g., building a tower together) with or without speech; or children may be playing with different but similar materials (e.g., one child eating pizza and one child eating an apple) and talking to each other about the topic.
Symbolic Play	Symbolic play is demonstrated when a child is able to use one thing to stand for another (e.g., using a green block for a frog). This shows the child's ability to create mental images.
Socio-emotional Play	Child engages in an imitative activity in which he or she fantasizes and acts out various domestic and social roles and situations (e.g., rocking a doll, pretending to be a doctor or nurse, or teaching school).
Turn Taking	When a child offers, gives, or accepts a play material to/from another child. This behavior must continue for at least two exchanges so that each peer both gives or offers and receives the item.

Verbal Socializations	
Initiating	A verbalization directed to a peer that is not preceded by another verbalization from the same peer within the previous 3 seconds (e.g., "What did you have for snack?").
Responding	A verbalization directed to a peer that was preceded by a social verbalization from that same peer within the previous 5 seconds (e.g., "I had pretzels for snack!").
Topic Maintenance	The ability to provide a response to a previous statement from a peer that is of the same topic or category as the initial statement. This should occur for at least 3 exchanges.
Conversations	Conversational speech requires the use of multiple, complex language skills including initiation and expansion of a conversational topic, establishing an interactive "to and fro" pattern of a conversation, and maintaining a verbal exchange.
Out-of-Self Behaviors	
Compliment Giving	When a child orients to peer, gives a complimentary statement (e.g., "You are a good drawer"), praise statement (e.g., "Nice hit"), or expression of reassurance (e.g., "Maybe you will win next time"). These statements must occur in the appropriate context.
Theory of Mind	A child demonstrates having a theory of mind when he attributes mental states (beliefs, intents, desires, pretending, knowledge) to himself and others and understands that others have beliefs, desires, and intentions that are different from his own.
Assistance	One child helps his or her peer by helping in getting up from the floor, completing a task, getting on/off play equipment, or responding to requests for assistance.

Selecting Social Skills for Treatment

There are several issues to consider when determining which social skills should be targeted for intervention in children with autism. These include:

1. determining the child's developmental level,
2. considering contextual and environmental variables, and
3. selecting skills that are adaptive and functional for the child.

The Child's Developmental Level

First, the child's developmental level needs to be established and taken into account. This is important in establishing which skills are appropriate to target given a child's developmental level. For example, it is developmentally appropriate to teach a one-year-old child to make eye contact or engage in joint attention; however, it is not appropriate to teach that child to take another person's perspective or to initiate and sustain a conversation. Therefore, it is important to reference normative developmental information (the age when an average, typically developing child achieves a certain skill) when deciding which social skills are relevant for training at a given developmental level.

Researchers at the CAC developed a curriculum based on typical development. The curriculum lists skills in the order that they would naturally progress in typically developing children. Once one skill is met, the next skill is introduced. For example, before teaching a child to engage in a reciprocal conversation, researchers at the CAC teach them to make initiations and to respond to the initiations of others. Then these skills are paired to teach the child to engage in a reciprocal conversation.

Contextual and Environmental Variables

In addition to selecting developmentally appropriate skills, it is important to consider the contextual and environmental variables that will influence the development of a skill for a particular child. It is important to select skills that are congruent with and respectful of the family's culture and beliefs. Different cultures, families, and professionals have differing opinions regarding what behaviors are appropriate for children and it is therefore important to determine the norms of a child's social environment when selecting and designing social skills treatments.

By considering contextual variables, it is more likely that the intervention and skills being targeted will be acceptable, feasible, and sustainable for the family and other individuals in the child's life. At the CAC, parents meet with staff weekly to ensure that they are an integral part of deciding which skills should be targeted in intervention.

Functional and Adaptive Value of Skills

Finally, it is important to select social skills that will be of functional and adaptive value to the child. Skills that are likely to be appreciated and reinforced by others and that will result in an individual's social and community adjustment are important to target in intervention. By selecting skills that are valued socially (noticed and reinforced by others), maintenance and generalization of those skills is more likely to occur. For example, if the child learns social behaviors (such as greeting others and taking turns) that will be reinforced after training has concluded, it is more likely that the behaviors will maintain across time and will generalize to other settings, behaviors, and people. The staff at the CAC ensures that socially relevant behaviors are being targeted by reading current literature and research and by continuously being educated and updated on developmental trends.

Assessment of Social Skills

It is important to assess social skills *prior to teaching* in order to identify specific deficits and *throughout intervention* in order to determine if improvements have been made. There are a variety of ways to assess social skills including through formal, norm referenced instruments, direct observation, and interviews or surveys with parents and other individuals in the child's life. Rather than relying on only one type of assessment, it is often beneficial to conduct several different types of assessments to fully understand an individual's needs.

Standardized Measures

One method of assessing social skills is through standardized measures. A variety of formal, norm-referenced instruments for measuring children's social competence are available. While some measures focus solely on social development, others are global developmental and adaptive behavior scales that also include a social domain.

The standardized assessment primarily used at the CAC is the Vineland Adaptive Behavior Scale (Sparrow, Balla, & Cicchetti, 1984). This instrument assesses development in four domains: 1) communication (receptive, expressive, written), 2) daily living skills (personal, domestic, community), 3) motor skills (gross, fine), and 4) socialization (interpersonal relationships, play and leisure time, coping skills). While each of the domains provides useful information regarding the developmental level of the child, the socialization domain is focused on assessing an individual's current level of social competence and areas that are in need of intervention. Information is obtained through a semi-structured interview with a parent or caretaker who is most familiar with the child.

An additional norm-referenced measure used to assess social skills is the Batelle Developmental Inventory (Newborg, Stock, Wnek, Guidubaldi, & Svinicki, 1984), which includes a direct assessment of the child via observations and tests. This instrument is useful in assessing interactions with adults, expression of feelings, self-concept, peer interaction, and coping in children from birth to age 8.

Standardized instruments such as the Vineland and Batelle Developmental Inventory are beneficial because they not only allow for an assessment of social skills, but also a comparison of children with autism to a larger comparison group—either typically developing children or the general population of children with autism (Charlop-Christy & Kelso, 1996).

Observations

An idiographic or observational approach is another method used to assess and analyze a child's social behavior. This approach is particularly important when assessing children with autism. Given that individuals with autism are a heterogeneous population, standardized instruments are often insufficient in identifying and addressing individualized social deficits. Observations provide additional information about a child that may not be assessed using only a standardized test.

The CAC uses a system for structuring observations that was recommended by Lovaas, Koegel, Simmons, and Long (1973). Observations occur prior to intervention and throughout the intervention process. Children are observed over a 40-minute period, alone and with a parent, therapist, and stranger who attend to the child and invite the child to interact. During four 10-minute sessions, various aspects of the child are observed. These include appropriate verbal behavior, inappropriate verbalizations, social nonverbal behavior (e.g., eye contact, gestures), appropriate play (e.g., pretend, socio-dramatic), and noncompliance. Through these observations, the child's behavioral repertoire can be identified along with any variables eliciting or maintaining the behaviors. These data, along with results from a standardized measure, then allow accurate planning of a treatment plan and outcome goals.

Data from Family, Teachers, and Peers

An additional means of assessing social skills is by gathering information about the appropriateness and effectiveness of current social skills from family members, teachers, and peers. Collecting this type of data is an essential part of assessment and is beneficial for two reasons. First, it is an important source of information when direct observation is not possible because of a child's age, lack of access to environments critical to the child's development (e.g., home, school, community), or the fear that observer effects will alter the child's behavior. It is also useful in that it supplements direct observation data by providing a more comprehensive picture of a child's skills and by validating the direct observation results (Kaczmarek, 2002).

Teachers, parents, and peers all provide information that may be beneficial in assessing a child's social abilities. Teachers have been shown to be both reliable and valid reporters of children's positive and negative social behaviors. Although few measures have been developed for teacher ratings, one that provides information on overall social competence is the Social Skills Rating System (Gresham & Elliott, 1990). Parents also provide useful information in assessing social skills, as they have a unique perspective on the social and communicative skills of children. Many of the social skills rating tools include forms that have been developed specifically for parents and also measure overall social competence. Finally, peers have additional opportunities to observe other children's critical social skills. However, most peer rating tools are focused on peers' perceptions of children's behaviors and social status rather than on ratings of specific skills. Regardless, information obtained from peers is important in determining the presence or absence of socially appropriate behaviors.

The CAC attempts to obtain information from several important individuals in the child's life in addition to doing direct observations and standardized assessments, as discussed above. Once a complete assessment has been completed and target behaviors are identified, intervention begins. Assessments continue to be completed periodically throughout intervention. Researchers at the CAC try to assess the child every four months or more often if needed.

Social Skills Intervention Strategies Used at The CAC

A variety of procedures have been used to teach social skills to children with autism. A majority of these strategies employ principles of applied behavior analysis. Those that are empirically validated and currently used at the CAC are discussed below.

Naturalistic Teaching Strategies

The difficulty encountered in teaching highly abstract and symbolic concepts, including language, conversational speech, perspective taking, and pretend play, to children with autism in highly structured settings has led many researchers to suggest that training procedures need to have looser stimulus control and perhaps be incorporated into the child's daily routine (Hart & Risley, 1980). As a result, alternative methods to the more structured teaching format of discrete trial have emerged that facilitate generalization, use natural reinforcers, and are easy to use by those who occupy the child's natural environment (e.g., parents). These techniques are referred to as naturalistic teaching strategies (NaTS) and include several techniques, including time delay (Halle, Baer, & Spradlin, 1981), the natural language paradigm, and modified incidental teaching. Each of these techniques incorporates three components and strategies: 1) motivation, 2) functional relationships, and 3) facilitators of generalization (Charlop-Christy et al., 1999), which will be discussed in detail below.

Motivation: In NaTS, motivation is increased by allowing a child to choose activities, by conducting natural preference assessments, by varying the reinforcement and interspersing the difficulty of activities or tasks, and by including obsessions as reinforcers (Charlop, Kurtz, & Casey, 1990; Charlop-Christy & Haymes, 1996). Researchers at the CAC conduct routine preference assessments with the children to determine highly motivating activities and reinforcers. Each week, the available activities and reinforcers vary so as to maintain novelty of preferred items. In addition, children are able to choose which activities to engage in and they have to negotiate with their peers to choose an agreed-upon activity. This allows child choice as well as teaching negotiation and cooperation.

Functional Relationships: A second aspect of NaTS that is implemented at the CAC is the idea that functional relationships will be more meaningful to children. Functional relationships are incorporated into teaching procedures as a way to teach a child to associate his or her actions with naturally occurring reinforcers (e.g., asking a peer for a car and gaining access to a car rather than receiving an arbitrary reinforcer such as candy).

Generalization: A final aspect of NaTS that is implemented at the CAC is incorporating strategies that facilitate generalization. These include using less structured settings, loosening stimulus control, and incorporating teaching into a child's daily routines (Stokes & Baer, 1977). The social skills group at the CAC takes place in a play setting (i.e., the playroom at the behavioral center or outside on a large lawn with a variety of toys and activities present) that closely resembles environments where children typically play. This naturalistic environment facilitates generalization and promotes demonstration of the skills learned in other environments with other peers. NaTS have been used to teach a variety of specific social behaviors to children with autism such as joint attention, gestures, and pretend play (Stahmer & Schreibman, 1992). These strategies are incorporated into the social skills group at the CAC to teach several skills, including eye contact, social initiations, joint attention, and turn taking.

Peer-Mediated Strategies

Early approaches to teaching social skills to children with autism primarily employed adult direction. However, a limitation of adult-mediated approaches is that they ignore the natural environment of children's social interactions and that social skills acquired through work with adults do not easily generalize to their peers (Rogers, 2000). Therefore, an additional or preferred method of intervention in teaching social skills is the use of peer-mediated strategies. These are especially relevant for older learners, as the presence of adults is more stigmatizing for children at older ages.

Children with autism are significantly impaired in the number of social interactions they engage in with other children (Koegel, Koegel, Frea, & Fredeen, 2001) and simply placing typically developing peers in sheer proximity of a child with autism is not adequate to ensure social interactions (Weiss & Harris, 2001b). Therefore, incorporating typically developing peers into intervention and training them to initiate, prompt, and reinforce social interactions will result in a more natural social environment and in greater improvements in the social behaviors of children with autism. Peer-mediated approaches have been shown to improve social interaction between typical peers and children with disabilities, including autism, and are therefore a common approach for social skills training.

Strain & Odom, along with their colleagues, have been a major influence on the progress in peer-mediated techniques (e.g., Strain, 1977; Odom & Strain, 1984, 1986) and have developed a model that is implemented at the CAC. A standard training protocol is used to teach typically developing peers to deliver specific social offers (e.g., invitations to play specific games) to their peers with autism. Peers role-play with adults until they have learned the strategies successfully and are then prompted to interact with the target children around designated play materials and activities. The typically developing peers engage the children with autism in positive interactions including sharing, establishing mutual attention, providing assistance, showing affection, and giving compliments.

External reinforcements (such as points or tokens) are systematically faded as the typically developing peers acquire the necessary skills. The typically developing peers who attend the social skills group at the CAC are usually friends or siblings of the children with autism who attend the behavioral center.

Video Modeling

An additional technique used to teach social skills at the CAC is video modeling. Video modeling is a technique that involves demonstration of desired behaviors through video representation of the behavior (Bellini & Akullian, 2007). A video modeling intervention involves an individual watching a video demonstration of a particular skill and then imitating the behavior of the model in the video. The target behavior is broken down into component parts and modeled by actors in the video. Video modeling intervention can be used with peers, siblings, adults, or the child himself as a model. However, at the CAC, adults usually act as the model in the video given the lack of frequent access to typically developing peers and the additional time that it would take to train them to act as models.

Video modeling has been effective in teaching a wide range of social behaviors to children with autism (Charlop-Christy, Le, & Freeman, 2000), including cooperative play, reciprocal pretend play, conversational speech, and perspective taking. These behaviors taught via video modeling were learned rapidly and generalized to untrained stimuli, settings, and people. At the CAC, video modeling has been successfully used to teach a variety of skills including turn taking, social initiations and responding, and conversational speech.

Scripts

Using predetermined scripts and script fading is an additional approach that has been used successfully to teach social skills to children with autism at the CAC. This approach consists of teaching learners to use written scripts or audio recordings that provide models of appropriate language. As the learners begin to use the scripted language in their interactions with others, the scripted phrase or sentence is systematically faded from beginning to end. For example, the child is initially given a written script with "What did you do today?" written on it. Gradually, the written prompt fades to "What did you," then "What did," and eventually to a blank piece of paper. The blank piece of paper is also removed before the scripted phrase is considered learned.

Scripts have been demonstrated to be effective in teaching several social skills, including social initiations (Krantz & McClannahan, 1993), bids for joint attention, conversational statements, and reciprocal conversations

(Charlop-Christy & Kelso, 2003). Each of these skills have also been targeted through the use of scripts and script fading at the CAC. This method of intervention has been easily implemented in the center as well as in the children's homes.

Self-Management/Prompting

Self-management strategies have also been used to teach a variety of skills to children with autism. Self-management strategies are focused on techniques that improve the social behavior of children with autism by having the individual keep a count of the number of times that he or she engages in the desired behavior or outcome. As long as the child achieves a predetermined number in a certain amount of time, he or she is given a reinforcer for engaging in the desired behavior.

Self-management strategies have been demonstrated to effectively teach children with autism a variety of social skills including eye contact and appropriate conversation, play, and responsiveness to verbal initiations. The CAC incorporates self-management procedures into each session by giving the child a card on which he or she places stickers for appropriate interactions and behaviors throughout the time at the center. At the end of the session, children are given individualized reinforcers for obtaining a predetermined number of stickers. This predetermined number varies depending on the child's current level of functioning and time in the group.

The self-management procedures used at the CAC provide children with fast and continuous reinforcement throughout their time in the group without interrupting the flow of the group or activities that may be taking place. Additionally, parents have reported that they have successfully been able to implement a similar system in the home.

Parent Training

Parent training is an important component of treatment at the CAC. Families are an integral aspect in the development and education of their children. Parent training with families of children with autism has been practiced for over forty years (e.g., Schopler & Reichler, 1971) and is now considered an essential component to treating these children (National Research Council, 2001). Research indicates that parents of children with autism can be effective interventionists for their child (e.g., Webster-Stratton & Herbert, 1993) and are able to manage problem behavior as well as teach several functional skills (e.g., Reagon & Higbee, 2009). Parent training has resulted in a variety of positive social skills outcomes, including increases in play-based social initiations, as well as increases in children's verbal and nonverbal communication skills. Teaching parents to implement behavioral strategies has also led to increased generalization and maintenance of treatment gains.

Case Study

Nicholas is a 7 year, 8 month old boy who attends the CAC's social skills group. He has been attending the behavioral treatment center for two years and was placed in the social skills group in 2008 after his needs became primarily social in nature.

When Nicholas was first evaluated at the CAC, he had several behavioral and social delays that his parents were concerned about. His mother reported that he would often withdraw during social interactions and seemed to avoid social environments. Nicholas also had poor eye contact and would avoid establishing and maintaining eye contact while interacting with others. Nicholas also presented as overly active and was reported to be extremely impulsive. While he had language well above 100 words and would initiate interactions or brief conversations with others, he would quickly change topic or walk away and begin a new task. It is important to note that Nicholas did have several friends; however, he would often become extremely upset with his peers, as he often misinterpreted what they said.

While at the behavioral treatment center, Nicholas demonstrated extreme resistance to social interactions with other children at the clinic and preferred to be alone with a therapist. He also was extremely resistant to non-preferred or novel activities and would often tantrum when presented with such tasks.

Nicholas made much progress in his one-on-one therapy sessions at the CAC. After approximately six months in the one-on-one program, he was less resistant to trying novel tasks and would tolerate non-preferred tasks with intermittent reinforcement. In addition, he began participating in social activities with prompting (board games, Duck Duck Goose, guessing games) that took place while the children were on breaks from the one-on-one sessions. He continued to require verbal prompts to make initial eye contact and still avoided maintaining eye contact while talking to peers or therapists. His tantrums decreased to only two incidents per month at the CAC, but his mother reported a higher rate of occurrence at home.

After demonstrating such success in his one-on-one sessions, Nicholas was moved to the CAC's social skills group, given that the majority of his delays were social in nature. The group consisted of four children with autism and three typically developing peers. The structure of the group remained the same each week but the activities varied. Nicholas's goals included increasing social interactions with peers, staying on topic during conversations with peers, increasing his understanding of peers' intentions, and making and maintaining eye contact with peers during social interactions.

After over a year in the group, Nicholas has made extremely good progress on each of these goals. He enjoys coming to the social skills group and has a best friend in the group with whom he frequently interacts. He is able to initiate and maintain a conversation for up to ten exchanges and will participate in conversations initiated by others. While he continues to make verbal protests when presented with non-preferred or novel activities, he will participate when asked. He still has difficulty maintaining eye contact for an entire conversation but will glance back and forth throughout with minimal prompting. His tantrums have also decreased and he has not had a single incidence in the past year while at the CAC. While his tantrums do still occur at home, his mother reports that they have significantly decreased and seem to be at levels more appropriate to his chronological age. Nicholas continues to attend the social skills group at the CAC and to make progress on each of the goals that have been developed for him.

References

American Psychiatric Association. (1994). *Diagnostic and statistical manual of mental disorders* (4th ed.). Washington, DC: Author.

American Psychiatric Association, (2000). *Diagnostic and statistical manual of mental disorders* (4th ed., text revision). Washington, DC: Author.

Bedell, J. R., & Lennox, S. S. (1997). *Handbook for communication and problem solving skills training: A cognitive-behavioral approach*. Oxford, England: John Wiley & Sons.

Bellini, S., & Akullian, J. (2007). A meta-analysis of video modeling and video self-modeling interventions for children and adolescents with autism spectrum disorders. *Exceptional Children, 73*, 264-287.

Charlop, M. H., & Haymes, L. K. (1994). Speech and language acquisition and intervention: Behavioral approaches. In J. L. Matson (Ed.), *Autism in children and adults: Etiology, assessment, and intervention* (pp. 213-240). Pacific Grove, CA: Brooks/Cole.

Charlop, M. H., Kurtz, P. F., & Casey, F. G. (1990). Using aberrant behaviors as reinforcers for autistic children. *Journal of Applied Behavior Analysis, 23*, 163-181.

Charlop, M. H., & Milstein, J. P. (1989). Teaching autistic children conversational speech using video modeling. *Journal of Applied Behavior Analysis, 22*, 275-285.

Charlop-Christy, M. H., & Haymes, L. (1996). Decreasing autistic children's inappropriate behaviors using obsessions as reinforcers with mild reductive procedures. *Journal of Autism and Developmental Disorders, 26*, 527-546.

Charlop-Christy, M. H., & Kelso, S. E. (1996). *How to treat the child with autism.* Los Angeles, CA: Claremont Autism Center.

Charlop-Christy, M. H., & Kelso, S .E. (2003). Teaching children with autism conversational speech using a cue card/written script program. *Education and Treatment of Children, 26,* 108-127.

Charlop-Christy, M. H., Le, L., & Freeman, K. (2000). A comparison of video modeling with in vivo modeling for teaching children with autism. *Journal of Autism and Developmental Disorders, 30,* 537-552.

Charlop-Christy, M. H., LeBlanc, L., & Carpenter, M. (1999). Naturalistic teaching strategies (NaTS) to teach speech to children with autism: Historical perspectives, development and current practice. *California School Psychologist, 4,* 30-46.

Charlop-Christy, M. H., Schreibman, L., Pierce, K., & Kurtz, P. F. Childhood autism. In R.J. Morris and T.R. Kratochwill (Eds.), *The practice of child therapy* (3rd ed.). Needham Heights, MA: Allyn & Bacon.

Goldstein, H., & Cisar, C.L. (1992). Promoting interaction during sociodramatic play: Teaching scripts to typical preschoolers and classmates with disabilities. *Journal of Applied Behavior Analysis, 25,* 265-280.

Goldstein, H., Kaczamarek, L., Pennington, R., & Shafer, K. (1992). Peer mediated intervention: Attending to, commenting on, and acknowledging the behavior of preschoolers with autism. *Journal of Applied Behavior Analysis, 25,* 289-305.

Gresham, F. M., & Elliott, S. N. (1990). *Social skills rating system.* Circle Pines, MN: American Guidance Service.

Halle, J. W., Baer, D. M., & Spradlin, J. E. (1981). Teachers' use of generalized use of delay as a stimulus control procedure to increase language use in handicapped children. *Journal of Applied Behavior Analysis, 14,* 389-409.

Hart, B., & Risley, T. R. (1980). In vivo language intervention: Unanticipated general effects. *Journal of Applied Behavior Analysis, 13,* 407-432.

Kaczmarek, L.A. (2002). Assessment of social-communicative competence. In H. Goldstein, L. A. Kaczmarek, & K. M. English (Eds.), *Promoting social communication: Children with developmental disabilities from birth to adolescence* (pp. 55-115). Baltimore, MD: Paul H. Brookes.

Kanner, L. (1943). Autistic disturbances of affective contact. *Nervous Child, 2, 217*-250.

Koegel, R. L., & Frea, W. D. (1993). Treatment of social behavior in autism through the modification of pivotal skills. *Journal of Applied Behavior Analysis, 26,* **369-377.**

Koegel, L. K., Koegel, R. L., Frea, W. D., & Fredeen, R. M. (2001). Identifying early intervention targets for children with autism in inclusive school settings. *Behavior Modification, 25,* 745-761.

Koegel, L. K., Koegel, R. L., Hurley, C., & Frea, W. D. (1992). Improving social skills and disruptive behavior in children with autism through self-management. *Journal of Applied Behavior Analysis, 25,* 341-353.

Koegel, R. L., Schreibman, L., Britten, K. R., Burke, J. C., & O'Neill, R. E. (1982). A comparison of parent training to direct child treatment. In R. L. Koegel, A. Rincover, & A. L. Egel (Eds.), *Education and understanding autistic children* (pp. 260-279). San Diego, CA: College Hill Press.

Krantz, P. J., & McClannahan, L. E. (1993). Teaching children with autism to initiate to peers: Effects of a script-fading procedure. *Journal of Applied Behavior Analysis, 26,* 121-132.

Lovaas, O. I., Koegel, R. L., Simmons, J. Q., & Long, J. S. (1973). Some generalization and follow up measures on autistic children in behavior therapy. *Journal of Applied Behavior Analysis, 6,* 131-166.

MacDuff, J. L., Ledo, R., McClannahan, L. E., & Krantz, P. J. (2007). Using scripts and script fading procedures to promote bids for joint attention by young children with autism. *Research in Autism Spectrum Disorders, 1,* 281-290.

Matson, J. L., & Swiezy, N. (1994). Social skills training with autistic children. In J. L. Matson (Ed.), *Autism in children and adults: Etiology, assessment, and intervention* (pp. 241-260). Pacific Grove, CA: Brooks/Cole.

National Initiative for Autism: Screening and Assessment. (2003). *National autism plan for children: Plan for the identification, assessment, diagnosis, and access to early interventions for pre-school and primary school aged children with autism spectrum disorders (ASD).* (Published by the National Autistic Society for NIASA, in collaboration with the Royal College of Psychiatrists, the Royal College of Pediatrics and Child Health and the All-Party Parliamentary Group on Autism.) London: Newnorth Print.

National Research Council. (2001). *Educating children with autism.* Washington, DC: National Academy Press.

Newborg, J., Stock, J. R., Wnek, L., Guidubaldi, J., & Svinicki, J. (1984). *Batelle developmental inventory.* Allen, TX: DLM Teaching Resources.

Odom, S. L., & Strain, P. S. (1984). Classroom-based social skills instruction for severely handicapped preschool children. *Topics in Early Childhood Special Education, 4,* 97, 116.

Odom, S. L., & Strain, P. S. (1986). A comparison of peer initiation and teacher-antecedent interventions for prompting reciprocal social interaction of autistic preschoolers. *Journal of Applied Behavior Analysis, 19,* 59-71.

Prizant, B. M., & Wetherby, A. M. (1990). Toward an integrated view of early language and communication development and socioemotional development. *Topics in Language Disorders, 10,* 1-16.

Reagon, K. A., & Higbee, T. S. (2009). Parent-implemented script fading to promote play-based verbal initiations in children with autism. *Journal of Applied Behavior Analysis, 42,* 659-664.

Reichow, B. R., & Volkmar, F. R. (2010). Social skills interventions for individuals with autism: Evaluation for evidence-based practices within a best evidence synthesis framework. *Journal of Autism and Developmental Disorders, 40,* 149-166.

Reichow, B. R., Volkmar, F. R., & Cicchetti, D. V. (2008). Development of an evaluative method for determining the strength of research evidence in autism. *Journal of Autism and Developmental Disorders, 38,* 1311-1318.

Rimland, B. (1964). *Infantile autism.* New York: Appleton-Century-Crofts.

Rogers, S. J. (2000). Interventions that facilitate socialization in children with autism. *Journal of Autism and Developmental Disorders, 30,* 399-409.

Rutter, M. (1978). Diagnosis and definition of childhood autism. *Journal of Autism and Childhood Schizophrenia, 8,* 139-161.

Schopler, E., & Mesibov, G. B. (Eds.). (1986). *Social behavior in autism.* New York, NY: Plenum Press.

Schopler, E., & Reichler, R. J. (1971). Parents as cotherapists in the treatment of psychotic children. *Journal of Autism and Childhood Schizophrenia, 1,* 87-102.

Schreibman, L. (1988). *Autism.* Newbury Park, CA: Sage Publications.

Sparrow, S. S., Balla, D. A., & Cicchetti, D. V. (1984). *Vineland Adaptive Behavior Scales.* Circle Pines, MN: American Guidance Services.

Stahmer, A., & Schreibman, L. (1992). Teaching children with autism appropriate play in unsupervised environments using a self-management treatment package. *Journal of Applied Behavior Analysis, 25,* 447-459.

Stokes, T. F., & Baer, D. M. (1977). An implicit technology of generalization. *Journal of Applied Behavior Analysis, 10,* 349-368.

Strain, P. S. (1977). An experimental analysis of peer social initiations on the behavior of withdrawn preschool children: Some training and generalization effects. *Journal of Abnormal Child Psychology, 5,* 445-455.

Strain, P. S., & Odom, S. L. (1986). Peer social initiations: Effective intervention for social skills development of exceptional children. *Exceptional Children, 52,* 543-551.

Vismara, L. A., Colombi, C., & Rogers, S. J. (2009). Can one hour per week of therapy lead to lasting changes in young children with autism? *Autism, 13,* 93-115.

Webster-Stratton, C., & Herbert, M. (1993). What really happens in parent education? *Behavior Modification, 17,* 407-456.

Weiss, M. J., & Harris, S. L. (2001a). *Reaching out, joining in: Teaching social skills to young children with autism.* Bethesda, MD: Woodbine House.

Weiss, M. J., & Harris, S. L. (2001b). Teaching social skills to people with autism. *Behavior Modification, 25,* 785-802.

4

Establishing Repertoires of Pretend Play in Children with Autism Using Video Modeling

Rebecca MacDonald

Social skills emerge very early in the lives of typically developing children. It is as if they are prewired to discriminate other humans from inanimate objects. They seek out attention from people in their environment and respond to others with focused and deliberate eye contact. *Social referencing* is one of the earliest social behaviors seen in young children. In the presence of an unfamiliar face, children as young as 10 months will look at a familiar adult, like a parent, for cues. If the parent shows disapproval, the child may cry or discontinue the interaction, but if the parent shows approval, the child will smile.

Joint attention is also an early social marker in young typical children. Joint attention involves an interaction between two people and an event in the environment. One of the first forms is responding to the social initiations of a caregiver. A child who is reading a picture book with a parent may look at pictures in the book as the parent points to images on each page. The child may then look up at the parent for approval or "joint" engagement. Children show these skills even before language emerges. The social response of the parent is enough to maintain this interaction as they read the whole book together. Another form of joint attention involves noticing a change in the environment and gaining the attention of a parent to "share" this event. Imagine that a bird flies into a window of your home. The typical child looks up at the bird, perhaps squeals with excitement, and then looks in the direction of the parent. Again, it is the reaction of the parent that maintains this interaction.

Social behavior of others serves as a powerful reinforcer for typical children; however, this is not so for children with autism. Children with autism who are faced with the same social interactions may look away or seem unresponsive to these social overtures. Play is one of the primary contexts for the development of social skills for typical children. Both interaction with toys and interactions with other people serve to help shape the complexity of play and language. Children with autism can lose out on those early opportunities to develop social skills if they do not engage in play with others.

Pretend play is one of the hallmarks of early childhood social behavior, yet children with autism rarely engage in play that has pretend qualities. Typically developing children tend to develop play skills in a sequence that builds on their language and knowledge of the world. Coincidently, play and joint attention emerge in the same developmental timeframe and both are linked to language in typically developing children. Deficits in joint attention and symbolic or pretend play have been identified as critical to the prognosis of children with autism (Kasari, 2002). Pretend play involves transforming objects or situations into make-believe ones. It has been postulated that pretend play or symbolic play serves several functions in typically developing children. It allows them to practice what they experience, to solve problems on their own and in their own way, gives them experience in mastering tasks, and allows them to experiment with new roles (Lifter, 2000).

Pretend play is characterized by a variety of behaviors, including using objects as if they were something else (use of play dough to make cookies), attributing properties to an object that it does not have (using a banana as a telephone), and using absent objects as if they were present (stirring imaginary soup). Interestingly, the taxonomies outlining the sequence in which children develop these play skills are the same across cultures.

Play in Children with Autism

Children with autism, on the other hand, tend to engage in play that is repetitive or stereotypic, and play that is indiscriminate or immature. Their actions with objects are simple and lack a symbolic quality. While typical children are learning to play by watching their peers, children with autism are not learning from these models, regardless of the density or frequency of these opportunities. These deficits are most apparent in the lack of spontaneous play.

Children with autism can learn to "pretend" to drink from a cup, or "pretend" to lick an ice cream cone through object imitation and discrete trial training, but this does not necessarily lead to their own production of untrained creative play with novel toys in new settings across different adults and peers.

Thus, the challenge is to teach these children play skills that will result in the emergence of previously unreinforced "creative" and spontaneous play.

Why Is Play Important?

There are many reasons why play is important to the social and language development of children with autism. First, if play has an odd quality to it, such as mouthing puzzle pieces, it sets the child apart from the other children. Second, if the child is unable to reciprocate invitations to play because of language or social deficits, he or she is less appealing as a playmate. In this case, it takes work on the part of a typically developing child to sustain the play, which makes play more effortful than fun. Finally, children with autism miss out on how children relate to each other, which serves as the basis for learning about cooperation, empathy, and collaboration. Play provides a medium for acquiring all of these social skills.

Teaching pretend play skills to children with autism has been related to improvements in both receptive and expressive language, thus lending support to the relationship between the emergence of play and language development. However, Kasari, Freeman, and Paparella (2006) found that teaching play skills may not result in a concomitant change in joint attention. Conversely, teaching children joint attention may not result in the emergence of more elaborate pretend play. While these two skills are important to a child's social development, they each require specific training in children with autism.

Building Blocks of Play

The building blocks of play are best summarized by the work of Lifter (2000). The taxonomy offered by Lifter is summarized in Table 1. Children first learn to manipulate toy materials in a simple manner. They learn to act on objects in specific ways, such as banging a toy hammer. They then learn how to combine materials to create something new, such as putting puzzle pieces together to make a picture or putting beads on a string to make a necklace. Once these early foundational skills have been acquired, children can begin to learn pretend play skills.

Pretend play involves a variety of skills that require children to use their imagination. Children can pretend to feed a baby doll, pretend that a block is an airplane, or pretend a small figurine is walking or talking. Pretend play can occur alone or in the context of playing next to a peer (e.g., parallel play). Children typically include some narration in their play. Pretend play also is thematic in nature and serves as a way for children to act out scenarios that they have experienced in their real lives, such as visiting a doctor.

Socio-dramatic play is arguably more complex and clearly more challenging to teach. Socio-dramatic play requires that children assign roles to themselves and their peers, share materials, take turns, and reciprocate verbal exchanges. Most importantly, it involves persistence or the ability to carry out a play theme from beginning to end. Examples of socio-dramatic play are preparing a meal using a kitchen play set, or pretending to put out a fire with a firefighter outfit and tools. Socio-dramatic play with peers is the most complex form of pretend play.

Lifter argues that teaching play using a developmental sequence will result in more rapid acquisition and increased generalization of these skills (Lifter, Ellis, Cannon, & Anderson, 2005).

Table 1. Developmental Play Assessment Play Categories (Lifter, 2000)

1. Indiscriminate act on object (bang toy)
2. Discriminate act on object (squeeze stuffed toy)
3. Presentation combination (puzzle piece in puzzle)
   - Pretend self (pretend to feed self)
4. Physical combination (string beads to make necklace)
5. Child as agent (pretends to feed doll)
6. Single scheme sequence (pretends to feed 2 dolls)
   - Substitution (pretends banana is phone)
7. Doll as agent (walks/talks for doll)
8. Multi-scheme sequence (feeds doll, brushes doll's teeth, puts to bed)
9. Socio-dramatic/thematic fantasy play (assign roles to self and others)

Teaching Play Using Behavioral Procedures

A variety of behavioral teaching procedures have been examined to teach play skills to children with autism, including discrete trial training, pivotal response training, and in-vivo modeling using play scripts.

Pivotal response training (PRT) incorporates the behavioral procedures of prompting and reinforcement with teaching procedures drawn from the developmental literature such as following the child's lead. Teaching occurs in a naturalistic setting using child preference during ongoing play to facilitate social interactions. PRT has been shown to be effective in establishing socio-dramatic play skills with adults and peers, and acquired play skills have been shown to generalize across toys and play partners.

In-vivo modeling using play scripts also has been shown to be effective in establishing socio-dramatic play with peers. Goldstein and Cisar (1992) used socio-dramatic scripts to teach typically developing children to engage in thematic play with a child with autism using three play sets, including a pet shop, a carnival, and a magic show. Teaching play using thematic scripts resulted in increases in theme-related social behavior for all children. Jahr, Eldevik, and Eikeseth (2000) found that when verbal rehearsal is added to in-vivo modeling children engaged in more sustained cooperative play. Based on these studies, modeling appears to be a promising procedure for teaching play to children with autism.

What Is Video Modeling?

Video modeling typically involves presenting a videotaped sample of child or adult models engaged in a specific series of scripted actions and/or verbalizations. The videotaped model is shown one or two times and then the child is directed to perform the scripted behaviors. Video modeling is emerging as an effective instructional technique to teach a variety of social skills, including play skills, to children with autism. Charlop-Christy, Le, and Freeman (2000) taught children to play games such as tag, Red Rover, and card games using video modeling. Video modeling has also been used to increase verbal statements during play with siblings and to teach children to initiate play with others. LeBlanc et al. (2003) used video modeling to teach perspective taking to children with ASD, and Scattone (2008) has used a combination of video modeling and social stories to teach social pragmatics in the context of conversations.

Video modeling has been used to establish complex pretend play sequences using a variety of play activities such as having a tea party, or playing with a pirate ship (MacDonald, Clark, Garrigan, & Vangala, 2005). Generalization of toy play across materials can be facilitated using video modeling. Children with autism have also shown increases in reciprocal pretend play with typically developing peers using video modeling. Children acquired sequences of scripted verbalizations and play actions quickly and showed an increase in reciprocal verbal interactions and cooperative play.

Clearly, video modeling is a promising avenue for teaching play skills to children with autism. Long sequences of play can be established relatively quickly using video modeling, and this training often results in generalization across a variety of materials, people, and settings. However, a limitation of these procedures is that children do not usually engage in spontaneous, untrained, or "creative" play as the result of video modeling. A variety of strategies are emerging as effective for expanding on the play taught using video modeling. Roberts, MacDonald, and Ahearn (2007) found that embedding a "substitutable loop" in the script increased the length and variability in play. Using this strategy, which is discussed further below, different characters were used across video models and characters were available that were never trained, which resulted in children using both trained and untrained characters in their play.

MacManus and MacDonald (2010) have shown that combining matrix training with video modeling can result in generative recombinative play across play set materials. These procedures are described in more detail in the section on "Strategies to Increase Variability in Play" later in this chapter.

Why Does Video Modeling Work?

Video modeling is based on the premise that children can learn through the observation of a model. Observational learning has its roots in Bandura's Social Learning Theory (1977). The elements necessary for observational learning to occur include: 1) attention, 2) retention, 3) production, and 4) motivation.

Corbett and Abdullah (2005) offer an explanation for how these elements are related to the unique benefits of video modeling for children with autism. *Attention* requires observation of a model and focus on the specific aspect of the model that is relevant. In video modeling, the video offers a restricted field of focus and therefore only the relevant features of the instructional model are present for the child to attend to. *Retention* requires that the child remember the model. In video modeling, there is repeated exposure to a model, both within a learning opportunity as well as through repeated exposure across learning opportunities.

Production is when the child actually imitates the behavior he or she observed being modeled. In video modeling, the child is required to imitate the model and practice these behaviors. This results in the behavior becoming well established in the child's repertoire. *Motivation* involves the concept of reinforcement. It is argued that the video medium is inherently reinforcing to children with autism and therefore children are more likely to watch videos and imitate the behavior seen in the video. A behavioral analysis of the reinforcing function of video modeling remains to be thoroughly explained.

Advantages of Video Modeling

There are many advantages of using video modeling to teach children with autism:

1. The use of video technology allows a teacher to demonstrate a model in a variety of settings that would be difficult to recreate in a classroom; for example, shopping at a store.
2. The teacher can prescribe and control the modeling procedures, such as showing a model from the point of view of the child. Then the videotape can be reviewed and edited until the specific desired scene is created.
3. Video modeling provides opportunities for repeated observations of the same model, therefore increasing the procedural integrity of instruction.
4. The edited video clips can be shown on a variety of media sources, from laptop computers and TVs to iPods, and can be reproduced to be used with many children.
5. As mentioned earlier, videos are often a preferred medium for our children, resulting in a preference for video instruction.
6. Finally, video modeling is cost effective because it reduces the need for teachers' individual teaching and efficient because children learn quickly using video modeling.

NECC Play Curriculum

Over the past five years, we at the New England Center for Children (NECC) have developed a comprehensive video modeling curriculum to teach play skills to children with autism. Using our knowledge of the emergence of play in typically developing children, we have structured our curriculum around four levels of play. These levels of play follow a developmental sequence. The curriculum is available to parents and professionals through a web-based product called NECC Preschool Playroom at www.NECCautismplay.com (see Figure 1).

The first level of play is *toy construction,* involving manipulation of toy pieces to create a new structure such as Mr. Potato Head. This level includes both simple construction and more complex construction tasks using K'nex. The second level of play is *toy play,* which involves a simple sequence of actions and vocalizations with characters or toys, such as making a sandwich. The third level of play is *pretend play.* At this level, children learn longer and more complex sequences of play that may involve talking for characters or pretending to be someone such as a doctor. The fourth level of play is *sociodramatic play* with a peer. At this level, children learn to take roles and engage in reciprocal social exchanges as they pretend to prepare a meal in the kitchen or order a hamburger from McDonald's.

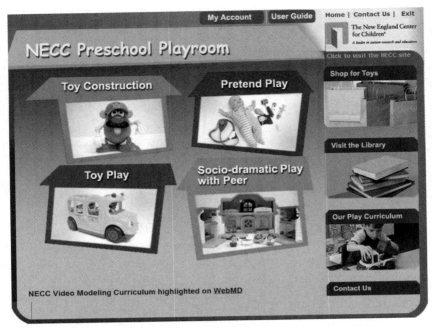

Figure 1. NECC Preschool Playroom Website

The goal is to establish a large repertoire of play skills with a wide variety of toys. Toys that are mastered through video modeling can then be played with in other settings, including home and the classroom. Children who progress through the whole curriculum are exposed to the major types of play defined in the play taxonomies developed by developmental psychologists over the years.

Teaching Procedures

The steps involved in teaching play using video modeling include: 1) developing scripts, 2) making the video model, 3) baselining performance on the play script, 4) teaching the play script, 5) evaluating performance without the video model, and 6) evaluating generalization of performance across people, settings, and toys.

Script Development

The scripts are developed based on observing typically developing children play. The children are videotaped playing with the toys for which a script is being developed. Then we watch the video of typical play and write down the children's actions and play statements. This information is then used to develop play scripts.

There are a variety of factors to consider when developing play scripts for a specific child (Table 2).

- The *language level* as measured by the child's mean length of utterance may influence the vocalizations incorporated into the script.
- The child's *fine motor skills* are important to consider in selecting materials to use during play. Large, chunky, easy-to-manipulate materials are better suited for children who have low tone or poor fine motor skills.
- Another variable is the presence and topography of any *interfering behavior* such as stereotypy or other challenging behaviors that may impede learning a particular script. For example, if Velcro is a medium that is associated with repetitive touching and uninterruptible rigid routines, avoid any toys with Velcro.
- It is also important to consider the *level of social behavior* already in the child's repertoire. Does the child have the skills to participate in play with a peer?
- Finally, consider the *length of the script*. Would your child do better with short scripts with a few actions and vocalization or does he or she have the skills to learn a longer play sequence?

You should modify the actions and statements made by the typical children to fit the level of curriculum that fits the child you are teaching.

Table 2. Things to Consider When Developing a Play Script

- Mean Length of Utterance (MLU)
- Fine Motor Skills
- Level of play (cause-effect, symbolic)
- Interfering behavior: stereotypy or other challenging behaviors
- Social Skills: solitary or cooperative play
- Length of script: Mastery of shorter scripts first, then increase length and complexity

The top half of Table 3 shows an example of the scripted actions and vocalizations for two typical children playing with a baking set. The types of actions include stirring, eating, and turning the mixer. All of these behaviors use the materials for play and are thematic in nature. Examples of vocalizations include: "First we need to stir it"; "Now we mix it"; and so on. Sometimes sound effects are paired with their actions. Typically, these vocalizations involve narrating the play that is occurring, and when two children are playing together they also involve regulating the play of their peer; for example, "Now we have to make something." The right column in Table 3 shows an example of a script we developed based on the behavior of these typical children.

Table 3. Example of Using Play of Typical Children to Develop a Script

OBSERVATION OF A TYPICAL CHILD		
Objects	**Action**	**Vocalizations**
		"Now we have to make something"
Bowl and spoon	Put spoon in bowl and stir	"First we need to stir it"
Rolling pin	Roll on carpet	"First we need to roll it"
Bowl and spoon	Put spoon in bowl and stir	"Now we mix it"
Scale	Pick up scale	"Now we have to look at the time"
Blender and bowl	Put bowl under blender and push blender down	"/vvvvvvvv/, ding" "It's ready"
Blender	Lift up blender	"It's all done"
Bowl	Pick up bowl	"Can I have all of it?"
Bowl	Bring bowl to mouth	"Okay thank you [slurp]"

SCRIPT		
Objects	**Action**	**Vocalizations**
		"Let's make dessert"
Rolling pin	Roll on table	"Roll it"
Bowl and spoon	Put spoon in bowl and stir	"Mix it up"
Blender and bowl	Put bowl under blender and push blender down	"/vvvvvvv/, ding" It's ready"
Bowl	Picks up bowl	"I want some"
Bowl and spoon	Spoon in bowl and then to mouth	"Yum-yum" "It's good"
Bowl and spoon	Put down	"All done"

Making the Video Model

When creating the video model, always videotape from the perspective of the child. Set up the materials as they would appear to the child when he or she begins to play. Begin videotaping with a view of all the materials from a distance. This can also include the person who is acting out the script (Figure 2, left). Then zoom in on the actual materials so that the child gets a closer look (Figure 2, right). If a main structure such as a barn or boat is used, the main structure is placed directly in front of the child and all other materials (figures/objects) are placed to the side of the structure. Many of the toys currently available make sounds. Be careful to remove the batteries so that all noises need to be generated by the children. Finally, edit the video and create a file that shows the full video model two times consecutively.

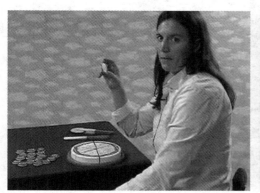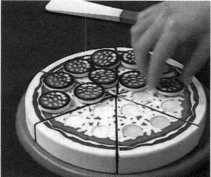

Figure 2. Example of Video Modeling Video: Whole Scene (left), Focus on Toys (right)

Baseline

Before introducing a specific script, take baseline to assess the child's current skill level. If the child already plays appropriately with the materials, then training would not be necessary. Set up all of the necessary materials on the table or floor (depending on the specific play activity and the individual child). Have the data sheet for the play script you are assessing available. Then bring the child to the toys and say, "It's time to play." Stand behind the child, being sure to stay out of his or her direct view. Do not provide any additional instructions or prompts and allow the child to play for between 2 to 4 minutes (depending on the complexity of the activity). Record the child's performance on the data sheet and determine whether the activity requires training.

Training

Many of the procedures used during training are exactly the same as those used during baseline. Again, print out the data sheet and set up the toy, then bring the child to the computer/DVD player and say, "It's time to watch a video." It is best to set up the toys near the video viewing area so the child can reference the toys while watching the video (Figure 3). Have the child watch the video model all the way through two times. Then bring the child to the toy and say, "It's time to play." Stand or sit behind him or her and allow 2 to 4 minutes to complete the play task. When the time is up, praise him or her for playing, regardless of how much of the play scenario was completed. It can take as few as three viewings or as many as ten exposures to the video model before the child will be completely independent.

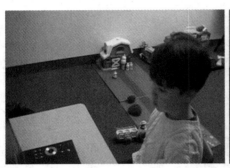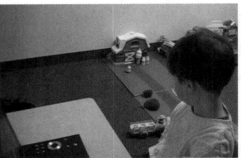

Figure 3. Example of Child Watching the Video Model (left) and Looking at Toys (right)

If the child makes errors on the same step three consecutive times, provide prompting using physical guidance only (avoid verbal instruction) to correct the error. Do not allow errors to occur more often, particularly in toy construction, as they will be more difficult to correct over time.

Mastery Probes

Once your child has completed the play scenario with 100% accuracy (toy construction) or 80% accuracy (all other levels) with the video, then present the task without the video. When the child performs at the accuracy level prescribed for that level on two consecutive sessions, he or she has met mastery criteria on that toy and play script. You can then have the child play with the toys with other people and in other settings. In addition, you can evaluate performance on the play script with toys that are similar but not exactly the same. For example, if you are teaching Mr. Potato Head, you might assess performance on Mrs. Potato Head and Carrot Head.

Evaluating Performance

To evaluate performance, data should be collected each time a session is run. Data are recorded on a data sheet that includes all scripted behaviors (actions and vocalizations), as well as the date, person who is running the session, and type of session—probe or training (Figure 4). While the child is playing, record a + in the box next to that behavior for each correctly per-

Figure 4. Sample Tractor Script Data Sheet

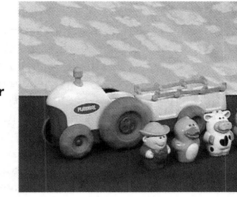

Tractor

DATE	
TEACHER/PARENT	
TRIAL TYPE (Probe, Training)	

Objects	Action	+/-	Vocals	+/-
Pig	Pick up pig		"Oink Oink"	
	Put pig in tractor			
Cow	Pick up cow		"Moo"	
	Put cow in tractor			
Duck	Pick up duck		"Quack Quack"	
	Put duck in tractor			
Farmer	Pick up farmer			
	Put farmer in tractor		"Let's go"	
Tractor	Tractor drives away			
Total		/ 9		/ 4

formed step in the sequence and a – for each incorrect step. Note that actions are listed on the left side of the data box and vocalizations are listed to the right side of the actions. These behaviors should be scored separately.

Following are guidelines for scoring play scenarios. Actions and vocalizations must be performed with the appropriate materials for them to be scored as correct. For example: picking up a cow and saying "moo" is correct, but picking up a cow and saying "oink" would not be a correct vocalization. However, for many play sequences the specific actions and vocalizations do not have to be performed in the exact order displayed on the video. Record each action and vocalization as correct whenever it occurs during the play session. You can score approximations or elaborations of the vocalizations within the play script as correct. You want some variation in the child's play. If he or she uses other characters or materials appropriately but not as shown in the video script, you should make note of this. Again, more variation in play is better.

Prerequisite Skills for Video Modeling

Several skills have emerged as critical prerequisites for learning using video modeling. Attending to a video and imitation skills have been postulated as logical prerequisites (Weiss & Harris, 2001); however, these variables have not been systematically evaluated. McCoy and Hermensen (2007) suggest that the length of the video may influence attending to the model, proposing that a shorter model may increase attending and therefore influence the successfulness of video modeling. In addition, memory could play an important role in learning using video modeling. Observing and imitating a model requires that the child remember the observed actions for the duration of the video and the period of time between the video and the task. In a study of more than 30 children, we found that the delayed imitation of actions with objects and delayed matching of objects to pictures were highly correlated with the ability to imitate an eight-step video model (MacDonald, Dickson, Robinson, & Ahearn, 2010). In addition, Robinson (2009) found that when children were taught these delayed matching and imitation skills, their ability to learn using video modeling improved.

We recommend the following skills be present in a child's repertoire for video modeling to be an effective teaching procedure for a child. They include: generalized motor imitation, attending to a video, 3 second delayed match-to-sample, and 3 second delayed imitation of actions with objects (Table 4).

Table 4. Prerequisite Skills for Video Modeling

- Generalized motor imitation
- Imitates actions with objects
- Delayed imitation of actions with objects
- Motor skills
- Picture to object matching
- Delayed picture to object matching
- Attending to video

Instructional Adaptations

Although the presentation of the video modeling script is usually all that is needed for children to acquire the play skills, modifications to the teaching procedures are required in some cases.

Prompting: Mazurski & Bourret (2007) demonstrated that learning occurred more rapidly when video modeling was combined with prompting. Prompting may be necessary to facilitate learning if a child is making repeated errors on the same step. Prompting or pre-teaching may also be necessary if a child is unable to perform one of the steps in the task because of his or her motor skills. For example, in teaching a superhero script with Batman and the Joker, part of the play involved putting a battering ram in the hero's hand. This proved difficult for a number of children and was therefore prompted.

In some cases, prompting only the first step in the chain can be helpful. For example, one student engaged in repetitive play during baseline and established a routine that he then continued to follow even during training. When prompted on the first step, he then demonstrated the rest of the steps in the play sequence. The addition of a reinforcement contingency at the end of the training trial may also facilitate learning; however, we have found this not to be necessary in most cases.

Segmented Video Modeling: Another modification that has been successful in helping children learn is the use of segmented video modeling. This involves editing the video into smaller segments. This allows the child to learn one step of the chain at a time. Tereshko, MacDonald, and Ahearn (2010) used a segmented video modeling procedure to teach children eight steps in building toy monsters using Mega Blocks. The videos were edited to show one step, then two steps and so on. All children were able to learn to build these monsters using this procedure. Interestingly, these children did not have delayed matching in their repertoire but were able to learn using a segmented model strategy.

Watching the Video While Completing a Task: Another modification is to show the video model simultaneous with the child performing the action. Ryan, Mahoney, Braga-Kenyon, and Kara (2009) found this to be a very effective procedure to motivate a child with autism to brush his teeth.

Video Prompting: Other research has suggested that video prompting can be an effective procedure to facilitate learning (Sigafoos et al., 2005). Video prompting involves showing the child one step in the chain and teaching to mastery before moving on to teach the next step in the chain. Video prompting would be an appropriate adaptation for play that involves motor chains, such as constructing a character with K'nex, or Legos.

While many children with ASD learn quickly using just video modeling, it may be necessary to adapt the procedures using the above modifications.

Teaching Using the NECC Preschool Playroom Curriculum

Toy Construction

Toy construction is the simplest level of play. Children learn to manipulate play materials in order to make new toy constructs; for example, using bristle blocks to make a car. This level most closely represents Lifter's early developmental play level involving physical combination of materials. Typically developing children often use manipulatives to create characters or structures that they then use in imaginative ways. For example, they might use interlocking manipulatives to make a pretend bracelet that squirts water. Learning to interact appropriately with play materials and create a variety of novel constructs from manipulatives is an important step in the development of play.

In this level, a child will imitate an adult modeling how to build structures using manipulatives. Toy construction includes toys such as Mr. Potato Head, K'nex materials, or play dough. The child must be able to perform simple motor imitation and be able to manipulate the specific materials for the toy you select.

Within toy construction, there are two levels: simple and complex. In simple construction, the child imitates constructing a basic play item. Simple construction typically includes imitating constructive toys where there are limited possibilities for incorrect responses, such as Mr. Potato Head.

Video Model: The video model includes a view from the child's perspective of an adult building the toy structure being taught. The adult models the construction at a slow, even pace. The video model is created so that the camera zooms in on the specific manipulation of the pieces. The whole sequence is shown, including playing with the toy once it is constructed; for example, driving a car that has been created from Lego blocks.

Performance Evaluation: In play construction, we evaluate performance using a task analysis detailing the sequence of steps needed to construct the play item. In Figure 5 you can see the task analysis for Mr. Potato Head. There are 6 steps in this sequence and they can be done in any order. Data are taken on the child's independence in completing each step of the chain. On the bottom of every data sheet there is a picture of how to set up the pieces of the play item, and on the right, a picture of the end form.

Figure 5. Mr. Potato Head Data Sheet

Mr. Potato Head

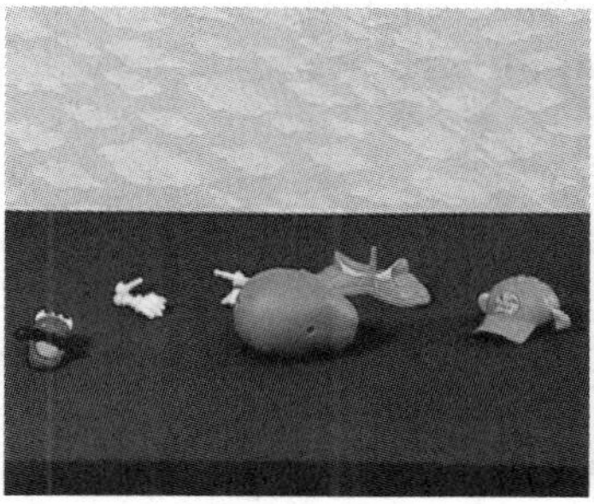

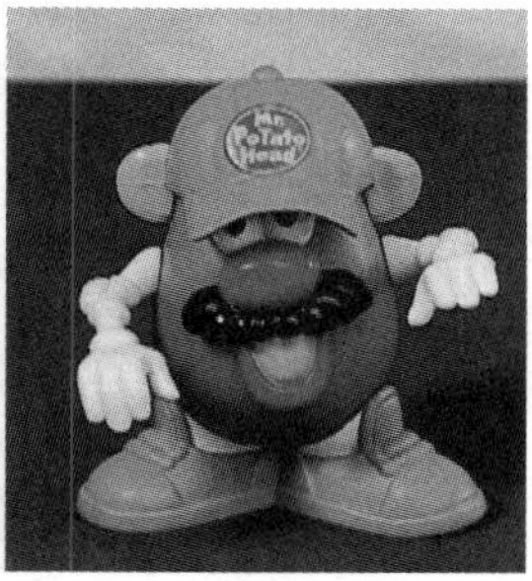

DATE	
TEACHER/PARENT	
TRIAL TYPE (Probe, Training)	

Pick up body						
Insert face into body						
Insert arm 1 into body						
Insert arm 2 into body						
Insert body into shoes						
Insert hat on top						
Make him walk						
Total						

Baseline: Begin by evaluating how the child plays with the manipulatives prior to training. Present the materials in an array on a table, including a picture of the completed toy structure, and tell the child to play. Allow him or her 2 to 4 minutes to play with the materials, and when the time has elapsed, announce that play is all done. Typically, children with autism may mouth the toys or manipulate them in stereotypic ways. We do not redirect their behavior, as stereotypy typically drops out once the child learns how to play appropriately with the toy materials. Observe the child's behavior and note on the data sheet any parts of the task analysis that he or she completes correctly.

Teaching: Again set out the materials in an array on the table, including a picture of the completed toy structure, but this time, have the child watch the video before he or she plays with the materials. Say, "It's time to watch a video" and have the child watch the video model all the way through two times. Prompting the child to attend to the video may be required. Then present the toy materials to the child and say, "It's time to play. Let's build a _____." Stand or sit behind the child and allow 3 to 4 minutes to complete the play task. If the child attempts to leave the play area, redirect him or her back to the toy and say "Let's keep playing." Record the child's performance on the task analysis data sheet. When the time is up, praise the child regardless of how much of the play he or she completed correctly.

Mastery Probes: When the child has completed the task analysis with 100% accuracy two times, have the child play with the materials without showing him or her the video. The child has met mastery on the toy when he or she is able to build the construct two times with 100% accuracy without the video model.

Generalization: If there are toys that have the same number of pieces and a similar construction format, you can probe to see whether the child can manipulate similar materials and create similar toy structures. As the child has more experience playing with the toy materials, he or she will learn to build a variety of structures using these materials.

Adaptations: If the child has difficulty following the entire sequence, consider reducing the length of the video model. As mentioned earlier, one strategy for reducing the length of a video model is to start with one step and increase systematically to the full chain of steps (Tereshko et al., in press). Another strategy is to edit the video to show blocks of three actions at a time. Once the child is independent with those beginning steps, then show subsequent steps of the chain. If the child has difficulty due to a fine motor requirement, you may need to select constructive toys with larger parts.

Simple Construction: At the level of simple construction, five or fewer steps are required to build the construct. The pieces should be relatively easy to manipulate and can include toys such as bristle blocks, play dough, and Mega Blocks. These typically require little hand strength and simple dexterity.

Complex Construction: At this level, more complex structures are created and the materials require more strength and dexterity to manipulate. K'nex toys are a good example of this type of play. They have a variety of different shaped pieces and it requires persistence and strength to pop them into place. In addition, they lend themselves to building a variety of structures. For example, K'nex Fish Eyed Friends is a collection of fins, tails, and ocean eyes that can be used to create many different fish-like characters. The set comes with pictures of different fish you could make. We use pictures along with video modeling to teach variations of toy construction.

More complex manipulatives often come with diagrams and pictures for the child to imitate. Ideally, children should learn to build constructions from the guide that comes with the toy, like the figures on the K'nex fish box. You can also increase actions with the object once it's constructed. This is easier to do when you have more materials. For example, in the Lincoln Log barn toy, once the barn is constructed, the horse can gallop over to the fence and eat the hay.

Generalization to Picture Activity Schedule: Once a child has mastered a particular construction toy, his or her play skills can be maintained through a photo activity schedule. A photo activity schedule is an effective strategy to help children sequence their independent play.

You can include a picture of the newly taught construct into a child's photo activity schedule. The child points to the picture in the schedule, retrieves the toy materials, and builds the toy structure without the video model. After it is completely constructed, he or she can play with the toy and then take it apart and put it away. Then the child moves to the next activity in his schedule independently. This is an excellent way to increase sequenced independent play and to generalize these learned play skills to home.

Toy Play

Toy play involves simple one-step actions paired with sounds or simple one-word utterances. Beginning play sequences at this level consist of five to seven simple/discrete steps. Each step is paired with a simple sound or word. Using a toy tractor, we teach a child to pick up an animal, make the noise the animal makes, and put it in the tractor (see Figure 4). With this type of toy there is little room for error because the child performs the same action with each figure (e.g., pick up character and put in the tractor). A sound is paired with each animal or character.

We begin with scripts that contain an average of five actions paired with very simple vocalizations and gradually increase the number of actions up to between nine and fifteen. We begin with simple sounds and gradually increase to three- to four-word utterances. An example of a more complex script is making a pizza, in which the child is the actor in making and eating the pizza (see Figure 6). There are multiple actions, cutting, putting on the pepperoni, and eating. Short phrases are introduced to narrate the child's play. There is a clear sequence to the play: make the pizza, cut the pizza, and eat it. The play also has a pretend quality to it.

Figure 6. Pizza Script Data Sheet

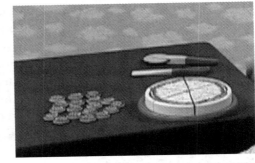

Pizza

DATE	
TEACHER/PARENT	
TRIAL TYPE (Probe, Training)	

Objects	Action	+/-	Vocals	+/-
Pepperoni, whole pizza	Pick up pepperoni, one at a time			
	Put pepperoni on pizza, one at a time		"Pepperoni"	
Pizza slicer	Pick up pizza slicer			
	Cut out one piece of pizza (two slices)		"Cut pizza"	
Pizza server	Pick up pizza server		"Eat"	
	Use server to pick up cut slice of pizza			
	Put pizza slice on table			
Pizza slice	Pick up pizza slice with hands			
	Pretend to take a bite		"Yummy"	
Total		/ 9		/ 4

In pretend play, two types of play are taught: doll as agent and child as agent, as described below.

Doll as Agent Toy Play: This type of play involves the child manipulating the characters as if they were animate. It includes walking and talking for dolls or characters. Toys that lend themselves to this type of play typically have figurines that can be manipulated. One example is using a Fisher Price airplane that includes a pilot and several passengers (Figure 7). We teach the child to talk for the characters as they board the plane and then have the plane fly. This involves picking up the characters, placing them in the correct seat on the plane, and talking for that character.

Child as Agent Toy Play: This type of play differs from the last because the child now acts on the materials as if he or she were part of the play scene. An example could include having a tea party (see Figure 8). At the party, the child makes the tea, pours the tea, puts in sugar and milk, and then drinks the tea. All along, the child is narrating his play with the tea set by describing what he is doing while he is playing.

Baseline: Again, begin by evaluating how the child plays with the toy set prior to training. Present the materials in an array on a table or floor, but do not include a picture of the play set. Tell the child to play and allow him or her play with the materials for two to four minutes. Observe the child's play actions and vocalizations and record on the data sheet. When the time has elapsed, tell him or her that play is all done.

Teaching: Again, set out the materials in an array on the table as in baseline but this time have the child watch the video before playing with the materials. Say, "It's time to watch a video" and have the child watch the video model all the way through two times. Then present the toy materials to the child and say "It's time to play with the _____." Stand or sit behind the child and allow three to four minutes to complete the play task. Do not prompt or correct the child in his play unless he makes the same error on three consecutive play sessions. Record the child's performance on the task analysis data sheet, and when the time is up, praise him regardless of how much of the play he completed correctly.

Mastery Probes: When the child has completed the task analysis with 80% accuracy two times, have him play with the materials without showing him the video. He has met mastery on the toy when he is able to follow the script two times with 80% accuracy without the video model.

Generalization: Generalization at this level of play typically involves substituting materials or playing with similar toys. In the pizza example, generalization is built into the play set because a variety of toppings are included, such as pepperoni, mushrooms, and peppers. Having a tea party is a more generic play experience, so present the child with a different tea set to see if he

Figure 7. Airplane Script Data Sheet

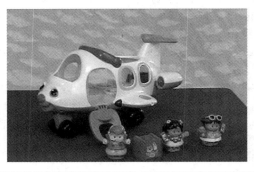

Airplane

DATE	
TEACHER/PARENT	
TRIAL TYPE (Probe, Training)	

Objects	Action	+/-	Vocals	+/-
Pilot	Put on plane		"Let's fly"	
Luggage	Put on plane		"Suitcase"	
Person 1	Climb up stairs		"Get on"	
	Put in seat		"Sit down"	
Person 2	Climb up stairs			
	Put in seat			
Plane	Close door			
	Fly		"Fly"	
Total		/ 8		/ 5

Figure 8. **Tea Party Script Data Sheet**

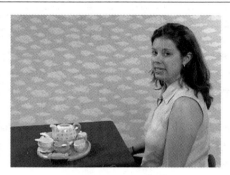

Tea Party

DATE	
TEACHER/PARENT	
TRIAL TYPE (Probe, Training)	

Objects	Action	+/-	Vocals	+/-
Teacup, saucer, spoon, tray	Take cup/ saucer/ spoon off tray		"I'll have tea"	
Spoon	Take spoon out of cup			
Teapot	Take teapot off tray			
	Pour tea into cup		"Pour it"	
Milk dish	Pick up milk dish			
Milk dish, teacup	Pour milk into cup		"Add milk"	
Spoon, teacup	Stir tea with spoon		"Stir it in"	
Sugar bowl	Take sugar bowl off tray		"Now sugar"	
	Open lid of sugar bowl			
Sugar bowl, spoon, teacup	Scoop sugar from sugar bowl into cup 1 time			
	Scoop sugar from sugar bowl into cup 1 time		"Two scoops"	
Spoon, teacup	Stir tea with spoon		"Stir it again"	
Teacup	Drink from cup			
	Put cup down on table		"Delicious"	
Total		/ 14		/ 8

or she can generalize the new skills to a similar type of play set. In addition, probe to make sure that the child can play appropriately with the materials in different settings, such as in his or her home.

The scripts at the toy play level increase in complexity from simple five-step actions paired with sounds to gradually longer play sequences that introduce longer verbal statements. However, play at this level continues to look very scripted. Although the scripts are based on watching typical children play, the scripts are still simplified. The goal of this level is to teach children to follow longer play sequences and to begin to narrate their play. This prepares them for the later levels of the curriculum, in which play begins to look more natural.

Pretend Play

Pretend play involves longer and more elaborate play sequences. Children learn to act out pretend scenarios such as a doctor well check visit, or a circus show. The scripts follow a story line and include both actions and vocalizations. They often include some type of dramatic problem, such as a fire in the building or a toothache. As described earlier, these scripts are based on observing typical children play. Both generic (e.g., a doctor kit) and unique (e.g., Fisher Price grill) commercially available play sets can be used.

Children should be able to complete all of the play scenarios at the toy play level and have beginning conversation skills in their daily speech prior to entering this level of play. All training and evaluation procedures are identical to the toy play level; the major difference is that the play is more complex, as illustrated below. Scripts range from 15 to 30 actions paired with 15 to 30 vocalizations. These play scenarios take longer to complete and provide more opportunities for extended play beyond the script provided. As with toy play, the scripts are organized by doll as agent and child as agent play.

Doll as Agent Pretend Play: At the pretend play level, doll as agent play involves the child manipulating and talking for multiple characters. Figurines such as Little People dolls take on roles; for example, the master of ceremony at the circus or the pirate on the pirate ship. The characters talk to each other, they move around a base structure such as the pirate ship, and they manipulate other materials, such as by driving a car or swinging on a trapeze. The storylines are thematic in nature. On the pirate ship, the characters are looking for gold using a telescope and a map. At the garage, a customer has a flat tire and the attendant changes the tire. An example of the circus script at this level is in Figure 9. We have found that children learn these play scripts quickly and are able to recall the play scenarios over time even if they have not had direct access to the play sets.

Figure 9. Circus Script Data Sheet

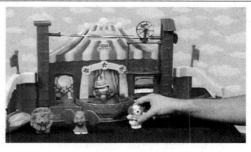

Circus

DATE	
TEACHER/PARENT	
TRIAL TYPE (Probe, Training)	

Objects	Action	+/-	Vocals	+/-
Monkey	Move through curtains		"Step right up to the world's most amazing animal show."	
Dog	Move to tightrope		"I'm Poofy the Poodle."	
Lion	Move to side of stage		"Roar."	
Elephant	Move elephant to center stage		"I'm Peanuts, watch me dance."	
	Make elephant dance by moving blue lever			
Monkey			"First, we have Lionie climbing the ladder to the high dive"	
Lion	Climb ladder		"Wow, this is very high."	
	Jump down		"Splash."	
Monkey	Kiss lion		"Great Job!"	
Dog	Move on trapeze		"Weee, this is scary."	
Monkey	Move to seesaw		"Now, Peanuts will make me fly through the air."	
	Fly through the air and back to stage			
Lion	Move behind stage		"I'm very strong. Roar."	
Monkey			"Thanks for coming to our show. Good-bye everyone."	
Total		/ 12		/ 12

Children's toys often come with a video of a play scenario using the toys. The characters in these videos are often claymation figures that talk and move independently and are animated versions of the toys. In a recent study, we examined whether children with autism were able to follow and imitate using these commercially available videos (Palechka & MacDonald, 2010). We developed our own videos in which an adult's hand moved the characters and talked for the characters using the actual materials that were available during play (see Figure 10). We found that two of the three children learned more rapidly from the instructor-created video. While the commercially available videos are an inexpensive way to teach play, they do not show the child how to make the characters perform the actions in the script. Having the adult's hand manipulate the materials may be an important feature of instructor created videos. We recommend making your own videos to teach play.

Figure 10. Instructor-Created Video Screenshot

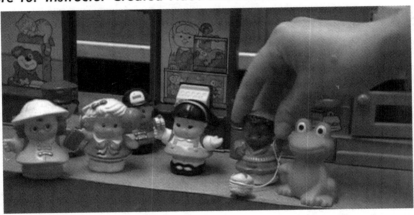

Child as Agent Pretend Play: Child as agent play at the pretend play level is most similar to dramatic play in that the children themselves take on roles and act out a thematic event such as firefighters putting out a fire. In this example, the child puts on a firefighter vest and a badge, calls for help using a walkie talkie, and squirts water on the fire with a fire extinguisher. The whole sequence is accomplished using a script that contains 17 actions and 16 accompanying vocalizations (Figure 11). Because we observed typical children play before developing these scripts, we are able to teach children the language of typical child play.

When developing a script for baking, we built in the phrases that the typical children used when they played with the baking set, as well as the sound effects and manipulation of the materials. In the doctor play script, we again included the language used by the typical children. Children with au-

Figure 11. **Firefighter Script Data Sheet**

Pretend Play Script

DATE	
TEACHER/PARENT	
TRIAL TYPE (Probe, Training)	

	Firefighter			Student	
Objects	**Action**	**+/-**	**Vocals**		**+/-**
Jacket	Put on		"I'm a fireman"		
Badge	Put in pocket		"Here's my badge"		
			" Oh no - a fire!"		
Walkie-talkie	Push button		"Come right away!"		
Mask	Put on mask		" I need a mask"		
			Breathing sounds		
Fire extinguisher	Hold fire extinguisher		"I need this!"		
Door	Push on door		"The door is stuck!"		
Axe	Knock on door		"Open!"		
Fire extinguisher	Pump		"This squirts water"		
Walkie-talkie	Hold to mouth		"It's big"		
Fire extinguisher	Pump				
Child	Jump		"Yeah!"		
			"The fire is out!"		
Mask	Take off		"I did it!"		
Total		/ 12		/ 14	

tism often require direct instruction in how to play with toys and what to say. We have found this scripted play to be an efficient way to give these children play skills they need to engage in play in a typical classroom or home setting with other children.

At this level, play may still be solitary or parallel. Just because children have the language and play skills to play with toys does not mean they will interact with their peers during play. This too must be taught.

Socio-dramatic Play with a Peer

Once children with autism have repertoires of play with a variety of different toys, they are ready to use these play skills in the context of their peers. During socio-dramatic play with peers, children learn how to assume roles and take turns in play. Using video modeling, we can teach children how to respond to their peers' actions and verbal comments, as well as how to initiate thematic play that is interactive. For example, when using a tool bench play set, the child learns to offer suggestions for what to build and to take turns with the materials.

When starting to teach cooperative play with peers, it is best to select a typical peer as a play partner. Our research has shown that using video modeling in which two children watch a video of two adults engaged in cooperative play has resulted in increases in reciprocal social interactions (MacDonald et al., 2009). Children learn to play with toys in a collaborative manner by taking turns, sharing, and working toward the same goal, be it pretending to make a birdhouse or to cook a hamburger on the grill.

Making the Video Model: The video model for this level is different from the other levels because there are two adult models, and the set up of materials is different because now two children are playing with the materials. The video modeling scripts are designed so that each child is assigned a character role; for example, in the airport video modeling script, the roles include

Figure 12. Tool Bench Picture of Adults as Models

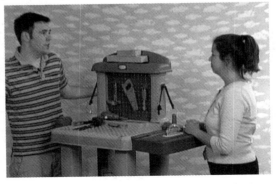

a pilot and a passenger. The video model is set up so that the adults modeling the play are on the side of the set that is associated with their assigned character role. Also the character or materials associated with their character are on that side of the scene. The models act out the script for their character.

The video model first shows the whole scene including both adults (Figure 12), then zooms in on the character who is speaking or acting. The actions and vocalizations at this level are similar to those at the pretend play level except now there are two people engaging in cooperative play with the materials.

Performance Evaluation: Performance is evaluated using a data sheet that has the scripted actions and vocalizations for both characters, as seen in Figure 13. The script for one character is on the left and for the second character on the right. Data are taken on the child's independent performance on each action and vocalization in the script. Data are also noted for each unscripted action or vocalization performed by the child.

Doll as Agent Socio-dramatic Play with a Peer: In this type of play, each child takes on the role of a different character as if they were animate. Now the children manipulate the characters so they are talking to each other and engaging in social interactions. An example of a script at this level is the pirate ship (Figure 13). The characters act together to find the treasure by talking to each other and helping each other.

Child as Agent Socio-Dramatic Play with a Peer: This type of play differs from the last because the child now acts on the materials as if he or she were part of the play scene. An example could include pretending to cook on a grill. The children take turns cooking and preparing the food, including turning on the grill, turning the burgers, and sharing the ketchup. The play script ends with both children eating the food they just prepared together.

Baseline: During baseline sessions, the play set materials are arranged as they are in the video model. The materials needed for each character are positioned on the side of the play set associated with each specific character role. The children are prompted to sit or stand in front of the play set on the side associated with the character role assigned to them. The instruction "It's time to play" is given, and the children are allowed to play for four to five minutes. As in prior levels, an adult stands just behind the children but does not give any additional instructions or physical prompts. This ensures that the toy, rather than the adult, controls reciprocal play.

Teaching: During teaching sessions, the materials are set up in the same manner as baseline, except a VCR is set up with two chairs in front of it. Children are directed to sit in the chair on the side associated with their assigned character. They watch the video model play script two times and then are directed to the play materials and told, "It's time to play." Allow four

Figure 13. *Pirate Script Data Sheet*

Pirate Pretend Play Script

DATE	
TEACHER/PARENT	
TRIAL TYPE (Probe, Training)	

Captain Script

Objects	Action	+/-	Vocals	+/-
Captain	Open gate		"I'm looking for pirates to sail with me"	
	Walk up stairs to landing		"Come aboard, Pirate"	
			"I should drive"	
			"I'm the captain"	
	Turn wheel		"Vroom"	
			"Arr. What do you see?"	
			"Fire the cannon!"	
	You drop the anchor		"Drop the anchor"	
	Point to map		"Let's look at the treasure map!"	
	Walk over to parrot		"Parrot, find the gold!"	
			"Maybe that is where the treasure is buried."	
	Turn Wheel		"Here we go"	
Total		/ 7		/ 12

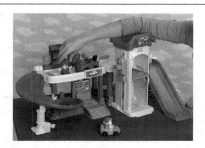

Pirate Script

Objects	Action	+/-	Vocals	+/-
Pirate			"I'm a pirate"	
			"OK"	
	Walk up stairs to landing		"Can I drive the ship?"	
	Sailor to crow's nest		"I'll look for other ships"	
			"A ship!"	
			"Over there!"	
	Get ball and load cannon		"1, 2, 3"	
	Jump on cannon switch		"Boom!"	
			"Aye Aye Captain"	
	Drop anchor			
	Sit in chair		"Wow! There is the gold."	
			"Let's send the parrot to find it."	
Parrot	Fly parrot		"Caw, Caw, Caw"	
	Land on white perch		"I see an island over there."	
Pirate	Hook anchor back up to ship		"I'll get the anchor"	
	Pirate to crow's nest		"We'll be rich!"	
Total		/ 10		/ 15

Figure 14. Boat Script Data Sheet

Boat

DATE	
TEACHER/PARENT	
TRIAL TYPE (Probe, Training)	

Captain Script

Objects	Action	+/-	Vocals	+/-
Man			"Let's ride the boat"	
Lady	Go to man		"Everybody in"	
Lady	Put tools under purple house		"I'll get the tools"	
Man	Put flag on boat		"I'll get the flag"	
Man			"The animals go down here"	
Lady			"Get the bear"	
Bear	Go up ramp into boat		"ROAR"	
Lady	Close ramp			
Man	Open green door		"Don't forget the food"	
	Put food below		"Here you go"	
	Close green door			
	Put on boat			
Lady	Get on boat		"Let's go"	
Boat	Drive boat			
Man			"Wait!"	
			"We forgot the _____"	
Lady			"Oh no!!"	
Lady	Open ramp		"C'mon _____"	
Animal	Go up ramp into boat		"Animal sound"	
Lady	Close ramp		"Now we're ready"	
Boat	Drive boat			
Total		/ 15		/ 15

minutes to play with the toys with the adult standing behind the children. No prompts or reinforcement are typically needed. When the time has elapsed, praise the children for playing regardless of their level of accuracy in following the modeled script. As in the pretend and toy play levels, once the children are performing at about 80% accuracy, have the children play with the toys without showing the video model.

Criteria for Selecting Typical Peers: We have found that selecting typical peers who have specific skills can increase the success of children with autism as they learn to participate in cooperative play (Table 5). Older children tend to be more patient and will wait for the child with autism to engage in the play script or will prompt him or her to perform the next action or vocal statement. Selecting a child who is flexible and cooperative is important. A typical peer who is assertive in play and who will engage in sustained attention to activities is critical because this peer will be facilitating the cooperative play. In addition, selecting a typical peer who has good social skills is important, because he or she will model unscripted appropriate social interactions and play skills for the child with autism. Finally, consider a child who is interested in helping and who is willing to participate in this new way of playing with toys.

Table 5. Criteria for Selecting Typical Peer

- Older than child with autism
- Flexible and cooperative
- Assertive in play
- Sustained attention to activities
- Socially competent
- Interest in helping; willing participant

For children who engage in stereotypic manipulation of toys, teaching play skills using video modeling can result in the development of a large repertoire of play skills. Parents often say they have a house full of toys but their child does not play with any of them. Video modeling offers an efficient and effective way to give children exposure to appropriate play with toys because children tend to learn quickly from video modeling. When selecting what to teach, focus on toys that are more generic in nature, as they lend themselves to better generalization. For example, most commercially available doctor kits include the same instruments but they might be different colors. Teaching a child with autism to play with a Fisher Price doctor kit should easily transfer to a different doctor kit with the same instruments.

Strategies to Increase Variability in Play

One concern in using scripts to teach play is that the scripts might interfere with the emergence of unscripted or novel play. Children with autism tend to learn the script and do not have the skills to extend their play beyond the script. There are, however, a number of empirically validated strategies available to help children generate more novel play following video modeling instruction (Table 6).

Table 6. Strategies to Increase Variability in Play

- Multiple scripts with same materials
- Extra materials available
- Substitutable loops
- Matrix training

Multiple Scripts with the Same Materials: The easiest strategy to generate more novel play is to teach multiple scripts with the same toys. The materials are the same for each script but the storyline is different and therefore the characters have different actions and vocalizations. Each script can build on the earlier script. For example, the first script might involve boarding the pirate ship (all characters start off the ship) and traveling to an island to get the treasure, while the second script could start with all the pirates on the ship and saving a pirate who fell in the water. Using this strategy, the children learn a variety of storylines and different ways of manipulating the characters or interacting with the toys. Given enough of these examples, children may start to generate new play.

Extra Materials Available: Another simple strategy is to make available extra materials that are never part of the video modeling script. For example, we have found that having extra toy food items available when teaching a script that includes a snack bar results in children using these untrained toys. Extra materials should include items that easily could be included in the theme of the play, such as foods at a snack bar, or vehicles at a garage. The mere presence of these additional materials can be enough for children to use them in their play.

Substitutable Loops: For some children, merely the presence of extra materials is not enough to generate novel play. A more systematic strategy for introducing extra materials involves use of a "substitutable loop" in which the script has a subscript embedded in it. This subscript consists of actions and vocalizations for which any number of characters or materials could be substituted. The video model shows several characters performing the substitutable loop, or using specific materials in the substitutable loop and materials are available during play that were never shown in the video model.

A simple example of this strategy was demonstrated by Roberts et al. (2007) using doll as agent play. A script was developed using a boat and animals (Figure 14). In this example, the script involved animals walking on a boat and included a loop that started with "Oh no, we forgot the _____," as indicated by the shaded boxes in Figure 15. Three animals were shown performing the scripted loop in three different video modeling scripts on alternate days. A variety of other animals were available along with the training animals, but these animals were never shown in the video model. Roberts found that the children played with all of the animals using the substitutable loop, even the animals they were never trained to use.

Figure 15. Boat Substitutable Loop Model

(Shaded boxes indicated trained animals and open boxes indicate untrained animals)

Actions/ Vocal in Loop	Sheep	Bird	Alligator	Giraffe	Cow	Dog
"We forgot the _____ "						
Walk on boat						
Make animal sound						

This strategy can also be used with the child as agent play. In this case, the child assumes a role in the script and manipulates different materials within the substitutable loop. Young (2005) used this strategy to teach ordering and preparing food with a McDonald's play set. She found that if the video model included ordering French fries, and chicken nuggets were also available in the fryolater, the children substituted chicken nuggets in their play. When using the substitutable loop strategy, it is important to find materials that could be substituted into the scripted play. Ordering different foods, or, as in the boat script, having different animals walk and talk, are some examples of materials that lend themselves to this sort of strategy.

Ostrowsky and Fouts (2008) used substitutable loop strategy to teach two children with autism reciprocal pretend play. Using a tool bench script that involved making several structures such as a birdhouse and a shed, they taught children to use a variety of tools in their play. In this example, two children with autism were taking turns, and playing cooperatively using the same thematic structure but varying their play within the context of the theme.

Matrix Training to Vary Play: The matrix model is a strategy for organizing the teaching sequence to promote generalization. This procedure has been used most often to teach language. MacManus and MacDonald (2010) applied this model to teach play to children with autism by sequencing the video modeling script such that play actions, characters, objects, and locations varied in a manner that promoted recombinations of play scenarios. Using superheroes (Batman, Spiderman, Robin), vehicles (batmobile, batcycle, batcopter), valuable objects (diamond, ring, money) and settings (castle, mansion, bank), scripts for three play scenarios were developed. These scripts were arranged in a three-dimensional matrix, as shown in Figure 16. After video modeling training using this matrix model, all of the children were able to recombine actions and vocalizations for the characters across combinations of play materials not shown in the video model. In addition, these children began using the play materials for novel play. While this strategy is more complex to set up initially, it has promise as an efficient way to teach children to generate novel play.

Summary

Video modeling is an efficient and effective teaching procedure to establish play in children with autism. Children who have the prerequisite skills of delayed imitation are ideal candidates to learn through video modeling. The procedures have been empirically validated with a variety of children, across a variety of different materials, to teach increasingly complex forms of play. Using video modeling to teach the play curriculum sequence outlined in this chapter, children can develop a rich repertoire of play skills.

Video modeling teaching procedures are easy to train and easy to implement. The most time consuming aspect of the procedure is creating the video models. However, once created, they can be used across many children. They can also be used by teachers and parents alike.

The emergence of novel unscripted play is slightly more challenging, but a variety of procedures can promote this type of play. The simplest strategies, involving multiple scripts and extra materials, can result in increases in the variety of play repertoires. Perhaps one of the most exciting areas in which video modeling has been shown to be effective is in teaching reciprocal pretend play with peers. Children show qualitative changes in cooperative play and social reciprocity in the context of play.

Figure 16. Matrix Model for Superhero Scripts

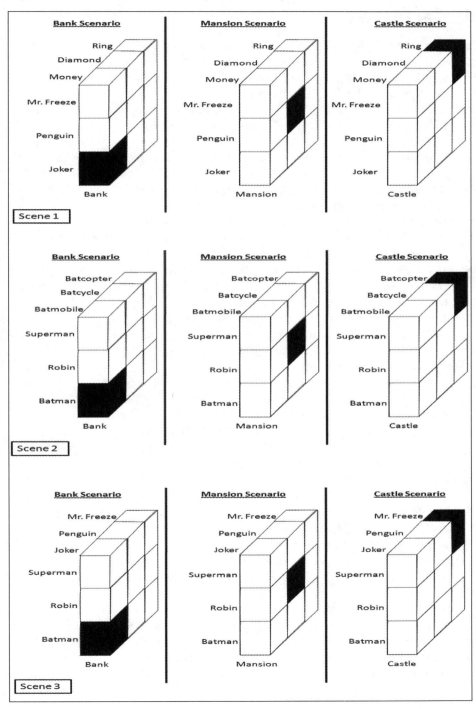

References

Bandura, A. (1977). *Social learning theory*. Englewood Cliffs, NJ: Prentice-Hall.

Charlop-Christy, M. H., Le, L., & Freeman, K. A. (2000). A comparison of video modeling with in vivo modeling for teaching children with autism. *Journal of Autism and Developmental Disorders, 30,* 537-552.

Corbett, B. A., & Abdullah, M. (2005). Video modeling: Why does it work for children with autism? *Journal of Early and Intensive Behavior Intervention, 2,* 2-8.

Goldstein, H., & Cisar, C. L. (1992). Promoting interaction during sociodramatic play: Teaching scripts to typical preschoolers and classmates with disabilities. *Journal of Applied Behavior Analysis, 25,* 265-280.

Jahr, E., Eldevi, S., & Eikeseth, S. (2000). Teaching children with autism to initiate and sustain cooperative play. *Research in Developmental Disabilities, 21,* 151-169.

Jarrold, C. (2003). A review of research into pretend play in autism. *Autism, 7,* 379-390.

Kasari, C. (2002). Assessing change in early intervention programs for children with autism. *Journal of Autism and Developmental Disorders, 32,* 447-461.

Kasari, C., Freeman, S., & Paparella, T. (2006). Joint attention and symbolic play in young children with autism: A randomized controlled intervention study. *Journal of Child Psychology and Psychiatry, 47,* 611-620.

LeBlanc, L., Coates, M., Daneshvar, S., Charlop-Christy, M., Morris, C., & Lancaster, B. (2003). Using video modeling and reinforcement to teach perspective-taking skills to children with autism. *Journal of Applied Behavior Analysis, 36,* 253-257.

Lifter, K., (2000). Linking assessment to intervention for children with developmental disabilities or at-risk for developmental delay: The Development Play Assessment (DPA) Instrument. In K. Gitlin-Weiner, A. Sandgrund, & C. Schaefer, (Eds.), *Play diagnosis and assessment* (2nd ed.), pp. 228-261. New York, NY: Wiley.

Lifter, K., Ellis, J., Cannon, B., & Anderson, S. (2005). Developmental specificity in targeting and teaching play activities to children with pervasive developmental disorders. *Journal of Early Intervention, 27,* 247-267.

MacDonald, R., Clark, M., Garrigan, E., & Vangala, M. (2005). Using video modeling to teach pretend play to children with autism. *Behavioral Interventions, 20,* 225-238.

MacDonald, R., Robinson, M. E., Dickson, C. A., & Ahearn, W. H. (2010). Prerequisite skills for learning through video modeling: Role of delayed imitation and delayed matching. Unpublished manuscript.

MacDonald, R., Sacramone, S., Mansfield, R., Wiltz, K., & Ahearn, W. H. (2009). Using video modeling to teach reciprocal pretend play to children with autism. *Journal of Applied Behavior Analysis, 42,* 43-55.

MacManus, C., & MacDonald, R. (May 2010). Video modeling and matrix training to teach pretend play in children with autism. Paper presented at the annual conference of the Association for Behavior Analysis, Austin, TX.

McCoy, K., & Hermansen, E. (2007). Video modeling for individuals with autism: A review of model types and effects. *Education and Treatment of Children, 30,* 183-213.

Murzynski, N. T., & Bourret, J. C. (2007). Combining video modeling and least-to-most prompting for establishing response chains. *Behavioral Interventions, 22,* 147-152.

Ostrowsky, D., Fouts, N., & MacDonald, R. P. F. (2008). Using video modeling to increase social interactions during play for children with autism. Poster presented at the annual convention of the Association for Behavior Analysis, Chicago, IL.

Palechka, G.D., & MacDonald, R. P. F. (2010). A comparison of play skill acquisition using teacher-created video models and commercially available video formats. *Education and Treatment of Children, 33,* 457-474.

Roberts, S. N., MacDonald, R. P. F., & Ahearn W. H. (2007, May). A method to teach varied play to children with ASD using video modeling. *Association for Behavior Analysis Special Interest Group Newsletter, 23,* 1-2.

Robinson, M. (2009). Training prerequisite skills for learning through video modeling. (Unpublished master's thesis).

Ryan, S., Mahoney, P., Braga-Kenyon, P. R., & Kara, L. (2009, May). Tooth brushing: Overcoming lack of motivation related to a task. Paper presented at the 35th ABAI Annual Conference, Phoenix, AZ.

Scattone, D. (2008). Enhancing the conversation skills of a boy with Asperger's disorder through social stories and video modeling. *Journal of Autism and Developmental Disabilities, 38,* 395-400.

Sigafoos, J., O'Reilly, M., Cannella, H., Upadhyaya, M., Edrisinha, C., Lancioni, G., et al. (2005). Computer-presented video prompting for teaching microwave oven use to three adults with developmental disabilities. *Journal of Behavioral Education, 14,* 189-201.

Tereshko, L., MacDonald, R. P. F., & Ahearn, W. H. (2010). Strategies for teaching children with autism to imitate response chains using video modeling. *Research in Autism Spectrum Disorders.*

Weiss, M. J., & Harris, S. J. (2001). *Reaching out, joining in: Teaching social skills to young children with autism.* Bethesda, MD: Woodbine House.

Young, J. (2007). Using video modeling to teach novel play skills to children with autism. (Unpublished master's thesis).

5

Facilitating Social Inclusion of Children with an Autism Spectrum Disorder

Saara Mahjouri and Connie Kasari

Children with autism face complex social challenges as they enter the mainstream educational system. The social climate present in schools can be difficult for these students to navigate, since a core challenge for autism exists in the social domains (APA, 2000). With the current push toward full inclusion, as mandated by the 1997 and 2004 reauthorizations of the Individuals with Disabilities Education Act and No Child Left Behind (IDEA, 1997; NCLB, 2001; reauthorized IDEA, 2004), children with autism have more opportunities to interact with their peers. However, inclusion alone may be insufficient for the effective integration of children with autism into the social networks of their typically developing peers (Burack, Root, & Zigler, 1997), and could even be to their social disadvantage (Ochs et al., 2001; Sale & Carey, 1995).

Parents identify social skills as the top priority for their child, but also voice significant dissatisfaction with the availability of school-based supports and level of attention schools pay to these issues (Kasari et al., 1999). If they can afford it, parents seek social tutoring for their children, usually in the form of clinic-based social skills groups. Several evidence-based social skills interventions exist for children with autism; yet reviews note that clinic-based social skills groups do not maintain gains over time or generalize to school settings. One reason may be that these programs are not *personalized* (Bellini et al., 2007). Group social skills programs have a particular focus (e.g., emotion identification or friendship development) and a set curriculum. Children who participate are rarely observed in their natural environments so that their social "personality" and particular skills (strengths and weaknesses) are unknown. The selected social skills program may not be a good match for the child's individual needs, perhaps explaining why treatment does not maintain or generalize.

In this chapter we describe interventions for children with autism that focus on their core social impairments. We note that one of the most striking aspects of autism is the variability of the symptoms. This variability has to be considered in finding effective interventions.

Early Difficulties

At young ages, children with autism seem less aware of their peers than children who are typically developing. Indeed, in one of the first published studies about children with autism, Kanner (1943) noted that Richard was "quite self-sufficient in his play" (p. 225) at 3 years, 3 months, a time when most children are interested in playing with others. Likewise, Virginia "sat among the children, seemingly not even noticing what went on, and gave the impression of being self-absorbed" (p. 231). Frederick actively avoided others; "when a fourth person entered the room, he retreated for a minute or two behind the bookcase saying, 'I don't want you' and waving him away."

The last thirty years of research have confirmed many of Kanner's original observations. The children Kanner described (as above) likely suffered from two under-developed core areas of development—*joint attention,* an early social communication skill, and *flexible social play skills.* Both of these areas of development affect the extent to which young children can engage with others in general and other children, specifically.

Joint attention skills involve sharing information or experience with others. These skills are shown through shared and coordinated looks between people and objects, points to share, and attempts to show an object or share an experience. These skills are different from requesting skills in which the child may use points and reaches to indicate a need or desire for something. Children with autism have less difficulty with requesting skills than they do with joint attention or sharing skills. They also have greater difficulty with initiating these skills than they do in responding to the gestures of others. Joint attention skills are communicative because they provide an opportunity to share something together; thus, young children may show a new toy to their playmate, or they exchange looks vis-a vis some event or action.

Social play serves a similar function. Play acts are characterized as functional or symbolic; children engage in play independently but they also spend large amounts of time engaging in play with others. Functional play involves using toys as they were intended. An example is when children play together by stacking large blocks on top of each other to create a tower with the goal of knocking it down. Symbolic play involves the representational use of objects, either pretending one object represents another, or attributing imaginary characteristics to objects. Symbolic play also affords children an opportunity to use language in situations they co-create with others (using language to demonstrate their imagination in the absence of objects).

Joint attention and symbolic play both provide an important developmental opportunity. Significant associations have been found between these early skills and subsequent language development (Mundy, Sigman, & Kasari, 1990), and later social interactions with peers (Sigman & Ruskin, 1999).

Assessments to Determine Early Intervention Targets

In determining appropriate intervention targets, structured assessments should be completed prior to beginning intervention, during intervention phases, and at the intervention completion and follow up assessment time points. Assessments should be relevant to the intervention. Thus, in targeting joint attention and play skills, we assess these skills in children prior to beginning intervention. The Early Social Communication Scales (ESCS) (Mundy, Hogan, & Doehring, 1996) are used to assess the child's initiations and responses to joint attention, behavior regulation, and social interaction. Total frequency scores are summed within each category, and these data provide needed information on existing, emerging, and absent social communication skills.

Similarly, in determining appropriate play targets for intervention, we use the adapted Structured Play Assessment (Kasari et al., 2010), in which children are presented with five different toy sets that can elicit functional and symbolic play acts. The child's behaviors are coded for frequency of acts, and the diversity of play. Diversity is the more important variable, as it yields information on how solid the play acts are within a level of play. For example, the child may brush the doll's hair, wipe her nose, and wash her face—three different play acts within the level of play referred to as "child as agent." Level of play (from functional to symbolic levels) is coded using Lifter's coding scheme (1993). Intervention then begins at the child's mastered level of play and works toward emerging levels. Establishing play level and using this as an entry into play interventions is important so that the child is not bored by play routines, and also not overly taxed cognitively by playing at too high of a level.

Another means of assessing joint attention and play skills is to observe the child interacting with a familiar play partner, such as a caregiver. These data can be important in assessing how the child engages with others, and also provides information on the appropriateness of treatment targets.

Interventions for Social Difficulties in Early Childhood

Early difficulties in joint attention and play skills require targeted interventions. Several single subject designs and at least one group design have been reported for targeting joint attention (Kasari et al., 2006; Rocha, Schreibman & Stahmer, 2007). One issue is that researchers define joint attention in a variety of ways and sometimes confuse requesting and joint attention; however, the definitions are clear from the typical developmental literature, and the specific difficulties for children with autism have been well documented (Mundy et al., 1986). Indeed, the skills that are the most difficult to change in children with autism are initiating skills (more than responding) and joint attention (more than requesting skills).

The methods used to teach joint attention matter. It is not clear that repeated drilling with little variation or drilling a skill out of context can lead to maintained and generalized learning. Because joint attention skills are used in the context of interacting with another person, *more naturalistic approaches are more successful.* In a randomized controlled trial, we combined a naturalistic behavioral and developmental approach to teach children joint attention skills or play skills (Kasari et al., 2006). Compared to children receiving early intervention services based on applied behavior analysis (30 hours per week) with no content in social play or joint attention, the children receiving joint attention and play interventions demonstrated greater skill development, and better language a year later. Most importantly, the skills taught in sessions with a therapist generalized to parents, and the skills maintained and increased over the subsequent year (Kasari et al., 2008).

Two additional findings emerged from this line of work. One is that the joint attention and play interventions yielded similar outcomes on language. A possible shared active ingredient of each intervention was joint engagement with the adult. Thus, it is likely that creating sustained joint play routines with the child and targeting skills within this mutual engagement resulted in greater skill in joint attention and play. Second, children with the least amount of language to begin with made the most progress in later language skills if they were assigned to the joint attention intervention. These findings suggest that teaching children at their developmental level (teaching prelinguistic skills prior to teaching verbal skills) is important to their later developmental outcome.

Mediating the interventions via adults may be a necessary first step for most children prior to peer-related interactions. Using a layered approach that involves developmental and behavioral strategies to target joint engagement, play, joint attention, and language skills, we have shown that caregivers can successfully improve these skills in their toddlers with autism (Kasari et al., 2010) and that teachers can facilitate change in their preschoolers in public preschool classrooms (Lawton & Kasari, 2011). The goal is that these skills will then generalize to their peers, although this has not been tested.

Peer-mediated interventions are accepted as the most evidence-based approach to improving peer interactions; yet, overall there are few preschool-based intervention studies. Over the past thirty years, only ten studies totaling 32 children with autism and 48 peers have been reported (Chang, 2011). All of these have been single subject designs, and fewer than half report maintenance and generalization data. Indeed, only one of three children typically maintains the skills learned via peers, with somewhat more generalizing the skills to a new context or peer. These limited findings may be due to poor implementation, as none of the studies report fidelity data.

Peer Engagement

A challenge for young children with autism is their lack of awareness of peers. For some children with little interest in peers, intervention with an adult may be an important first step prior to moving to peer interactions. For other children, peer-mediated interventions may be successful in helping to socialize and bring them into interaction with others.

The heterogeneity of the autism disorder suggests that a single intervention will not be effective with *all* children; thus, it will be important to have a means for assessing child strengths and weaknesses that will lead to effective social interventions. A child's "social personality" may provide important information about potential effective interventions. Wing and Gould (1979) provided such a categorization framework of children's social differences, ranging from *socially aloof and indifferent* to *passive* to other's attempts to engage them to *active but odd*—the child has social interest but is mostly inappropriate. Some children are expected to have *appropriate social interest and interaction.*

It may be that for aloof and indifferent children, a peer-mediated intervention will be more effective because the motivation for social engagement will not occur without active involvement of other children. For children who are aware of social relationships but do not have the skills to engage in them appropriately, direct instruction with the child with autism may be more effective because the child may have enough awareness and motivation to change his or her behavior.

A number of programs that provide children direct instruction of social skills are available. However, one issue is that most programs do not individualize instruction to the participant; thus, the social personality of the child is not considered. Another issue is that children are often unacquainted with each other. That is, most come from different schools or classrooms, so that skills learned in the group cannot be easily maintained with the same peers. Thus, while these programs have shown change in individual child outcomes, they tend not to maintain and generalize to other contexts, such as the school.

Another issue concerns how change in social skills is measured. While there is agreement that certain skills (i.e., greetings, eye contact, conversation skills) constitute necessary social competencies, the efficacy of specific treatments cannot be compared, without agreement upon the necessary skill outcomes. The variability in outcome measures makes it difficult to make reasonable comparisons across studies. Many studies have relied on rating social skills before and after treatment. However, the evaluation of change has often been obtained from informants who may or may not have access to observed differences in the children (e.g., parents are asked to evaluate social skills at school but may not be present at school). Or the informant is actively involved in the treatment and thus may be biased (e.g., parent mediated intervention in which parents also report on change in the children). One solution to these issues is to use multiple informants (parents, teachers, peers, self-report) and to use observers of children in natural settings who are also blind to treatment condition.

Assessment to Inform Social Skills Intervention

Examining the level of social interactions a child is having without intervention can inform the specific targets of social skills intervention. As autism is highly variable, it is important to assess each child's social personality. Is the child aware of others, actively attempting to engage but going about it oddly or aggresively? Or is the child happy on his or her own, appearing socially aloof? Most social skills programs do not do in-depth assessments prior to beginning treatment. One goal of future intervention studies is to assess child behavior using a variety of direct observations and reports from informed others. This information should provide details about the child's social skills across a variety of contexts. Interventions targeted to the child's particular set of social strengths and weaknesses should translate to greater maintenance and generalization of social skills, a persistent limitation in current intervention studies.

Depending on the focus of the intervention, outcome measures should link to the intervention content. Thus, if the goal is to increase engagement with peers during playground time at school, an outcome measure should be observations of playground behavior at school. Similarly, if the focus is on friendship development, reports of friendship reciprocity, and friendship quality from the target child and his or her nominated friends should be obtained.

Social Skills Intervention Research

Most social skills intervention programs use adults to deliver social skills information to children with ASD. Children may practice their skills with other children in the group, but the actual information often comes from the adult leader. Outcome measures are often rating scales of whether there has been an improvement in social skills, and raters are often the group leaders, or the parents. Sometimes the child with ASD is also tested for increases in his or her social knowledge using paper and pencil tests.

Few studies of school-aged children with autism have used peers as mediators of social skills interventions. Trained peers can be important change agents since they can increase the dose of intervention delivered to children with autism throughout the school day. When peers deliver the intervention, the outcomes are typically observational measures, and the study designs are overwhelmingly single subject designs (Chang, 2011). Kasari et al. (2011) implemented a randomized controlled trial in schools that compared peer mediated versus child assisted (1:1 adult-mediated) interventions and found several positive changes for children who received the peer interventions. In this study, outcome measures included observations as well as self and other reports (peers and teachers). At the end of treatment, children with autism receiving peer interventions were identified by more peers as friends, were observed to spend more social time (e.g., recess) engaged with peers, and were perceived by their classmates as being more socially connected. Teachers also noted improvements in the social skills of children randomized to the peer condition.

Similarly, Bauminger (2002) found that her peer-mediated, school-based intervention resulted in increased peer interaction and decreased isolation. The findings of these studies highlight two important elements in social skills interventions. First, the shift toward using peers in a naturalistic environment, rather than teaching discrete skills in isolation, may have better results in generalizing to the school environment. Second, measuring increased friendships and social time engaged appear to be important outcome measures that may be more telling about children's social experience than measuring specific skill knowledge.

Unfortunately, few studies have examined the effects of social skills interventions delivered in the school environment. Several practices have emerged successful; however, they often lack the empirical evidence needed for widespread dissemination. School-based interventions are difficult to implement, given the abundance of obstacles presented by school systems. It is often difficult to randomize children to treatment and no treatment groups, as schools will not agree to withhold treatment. Further, the school environment presents several uncontrollable factors, potentially rendering the fidelity of intervention and delivery and quality of data collection less than desired. These practical difficulties help explain the current gap between research and practice.

Practical Suggestions for Social Skills Interventions in School

Informed by current research, assessment, and observations of children in the school setting, a few consistent recommendations for improving social skills in children with ASDs have emerged. The following section identifies why school is an important setting for intervention, then describes a few guiding principles for implementing social skills intervention in primary aged children.

School-based Treatments: Schools provide a rich social environment, fraught with different demands and pressures. Bringing a model of social skills treatment into schools is recommended for intervention efforts. All students can benefit from school-based social skills training. Further, by teaching skills in the context that they are usually encountered, students are more likely to generalize skills taught by practicing them in a relevant environment. Friendships developed in school groups may also better generalize to other social settings in school.

Strategy #1: Facilitate Engaging Social Play on the Schoolyard

Recess is a very important part of the school day for children. For many, it is one of the only times to connect with friends, as well as to get energy out in a productive manner. Unfortunately, children with ASDs can be overwhelmed with the social expectations of the playground and the excessive sensory stimuli. Many may not know how to join in games, or cannot respond appropriately to the rules and structure of games. These behaviors can result in stigmatization or a preference for social isolation. Therefore, it is hypothesized that an effective social skills intervention at school will incorporate generalizing to the playground. Adults (school personnel and clinicians) should be trained and supported to look for kids who are isolated and encourage them to participate in games, use peers to redirect negative or isolating social behaviors, create fun and engaging games that encourage participation by all children, and fade out once children are in a sustainable level of play.

Key components: positive affect and enthusiasm from adults facilitating intervention. A high level of cooperation and investment from school personnel. Adequate supplies, play areas, and supervision.

Positive group leader qualities: flexible, creative, energetic, and playful. The ability to communicate effectively with all adults (teachers, aides, administrators, parents) in the school environment.

Strategy #2: Engineering Social Experiences with Peers

For many children with ASDs, the intrinsic reward of social interaction is not strong enough for them to initiate interactions with peers. Therefore, it is important to examine their specific interests, and create social opportunities around shared interests for children. Any structured activities or clubs that focus on activities children normally enjoy can provide a rich environment to practice social skills and foster friendships.

Often, children with ASDs do not have the social acuity to seek out and identify peers with similar interests, and therefore they have difficulty developing their social niche. Schools can play an important role, by providing the environment and clinician or school personnel support to create social groups where kids participate in activities they enjoy, and improve social skills and increase friendships as a byproduct.

Key components: school culture promoting the involvement of peers. Teacher and parental involvement in identifying supportive peers. Creativity in determining activities to capture the interest of children and peers.

Social activity ideas: playground games that are varied and age appropriate. Some examples are: cooking class, LEGO ™ or Puzzle club, video game tournament, filmmaking group, drama games, or a movie club.

Strategy #3: Sequential Interventions to Account for the Variability of Symptoms

A primary struggle in implementing social skills interventions is that a "one size fits all" approach is simply not sufficient for the variability that autism spectrum disorders present. Some children may benefit from specific skill instruction, whereas others may need practice interacting with peers in socially acceptable ways.

In order for a successful social skills treatment to account for the various needs of children, it is important to first instruct the child in skills necessary for social interaction, and then create and facilitate social opportunities for students to practice these skills with peers in naturalistic settings. In order for social skills treatments to be effective, both of these areas must be addressed and intervention maintenance should occur. For example, a child may be instructed in how to join a game in a small group, and then supported in joining a group of peers to play the game. Once the child has sufficiently shown the ability to interact with peers, clinicians or school personnel should be available to provide additional social coaching, as needed.

Key components: specific assessment to determine intervention targets. Flexible timeline for completion. Long-term investment from parents and schools to follow through and maintain social supports.

Active ingredients of sequence: 1) Priming a skill in young children using behavioral strategies, and then 2) Using more developmental and naturalistic strategies to help solidify the skill. (Example is the study by Kasari et al., 2006, in which brief discrete trial training was used prior to milieu play episodes to teach joint attention or play skills.) 3) Reassessing children's social needs through development, to determine the need for increased/decreased intensity and follow up.

A practical example of a sequential intervention approach is to break down skills needed in separate sets such as below:

1. *Instruct skill → accepting the rules of a game and being a good winner/loser.*
2. *Priming activity → practice game of handball in classroom, with group members. Positive feedback for turn-taking, and responding appropriately to winning/losing.*
3. *Supported activity → with adult support, join recess game of handball with trained peers. Adult feedback, when positive skills are displayed, to all children involved.*
4. *Generalization → children with ASDs are encouraged to join in a game, general adult supervision to ensure no children are isolated.*

Support Throughout the Life Course

Thus far, the issues this chapter has addressed are pertinent to early childhood and primary aged children. Unfortunately, the difficulty children with autism have in developing and maintaining positive peer relationships and friendships continues well into adulthood. Orsmond, Krauss, and Seltzer (2004) asked 235 parents about the peer relations of their adolescent and adult children with autism. Almost half reported no peer relationships at all. Likewise, Howlin and colleagues (2004) found that 56% of 68 adults with autism reported no friends or acquaintances. Additionally, school inclusion with typical age mates was not associated with having peer relationships. Thus, an individual's participation in an inclusive setting did not result in a greater chance of having a friend.

Some models to improve social competency in adolescents incorporate parents as part of the treatment (Laugeson, Frankel, Mogil, & Dillon, 2008). In the social skills program (PEERS) of Laugeson and colleagues, teenagers are instructed on positive and relevant social etiquette. For example, one session focuses on the differences in communication etiquette via e-mail versus the telephone. Additionally, teenagers in the group are encouraged to have social gatherings as homework. This aspect is aimed to improve generalization, as the groups are conducted in clinical settings. Concurrently, parents attend informational sessions instructing them on the best ways to support the social skill development in their teenager. After the intervention/parent sessions, teenagers and parents are briefed on what each covered. This aspect of simultaneous treatment of both the adolescent and their parents seems likely to influence long-term change.

Adolescents are a difficult group for which to design and implement effective social skills interventions. Research has indicated that adolescents with high functioning autism are aware of their difficulties in peer interactions. It stands to reason that their heightened awareness of their social status would result in increased sensitivity. This should be taken into account when developing interventions. Adolescents with ASDs were also found to experience higher levels of loneliness than their typical peers (Locke et al., 2010). Perhaps an effective approach to improving social skills for this age group would include activities that the adolescents naturally enjoy or are interested in. Project-based groups can teach social skills, teamwork, and cooperation, all while providing enrichment. Projects can also include community service activities. This can intensify the benefit of social skills programs for society. Not only are adolescents improving their skills, they are becoming more engaged with their peers, and visible and connected to their communities.

Conclusions

In the case of autism, no single intervention will suffice. If children are to build social competency, then intervention efforts must address the variability of the disorder itself. Given the success of interventions such as those by Barry et al. (2003) and Bauminger (2002), peer-mediated models are necessary to promote the generalization of social skills across different contexts of a child with autism's life. Additionally, both in the early joint attention and symbolic play interventions and adolescent social skills groups, parents and caregivers are a necessary component of successful intervention implementation. It is recommended to provide intervention efforts throughout the developmental trajectory, targeting different aspects of the core deficits of autism. Additionally, it is necessary to include all members of the child with autism's social network (e.g., parents, school, and community).

Child: Change begins with the child. The child is the primary target of any intervention, be it early communication or social skills and engagement. The most intense intervention efforts must be directed towards the child. In early childhood, interventions targeting joint attention and symbolic play skills can foster and support communication and language development. Once those abilities are adequately developed, social skills training programs in naturalistic settings can improve the child's behaviors that enable him or her to engage with peers. Through adolescence, the target of intervention must continue to build and develop these skills. Adolescents must be taught to functionally transfer early developed social competence into behaviors that allow them to interact with their peer group.

Family: Parents, family members, and anyone involved in the child's home life are an integral part of catalyzing and sustaining positive change. Parents are involved in implementing and supporting intervention directly in early childhood and indirectly in childhood through adolescence. For any intervention effects to be lasting, people in the child's home must continue to foster an environment that supports the child and his or her newly acquired skills. Improved communication, language, and social behaviors can improve family relationships. They can also reduce caregiver stress.

School: Once children have developed early competencies that have been supported in their home life, they can enter school with improved social abilities. These skills will allow them to fully benefit from inclusive opportunities. Additionally, interventions targeting social interactions, conducted in a school environment, increase the ability to generalize skills. Members of the school community must be supported to facilitate positive interactions between peers, so that everyone in the school environment can grow as a result of the experience.

Community: There is less evidence for community involvement in the positive social development of children with autism. It stands to reason, however, that once these children are supported to become contributing members of society, communities will benefit. Additionally, any intervention efforts targeted toward adolescents can incorporate community service components. Thus, adolescents have a shared cause to work toward, and practice their social skills.

When conceptualizing and implementing social skills interventions, researchers and practitioners are urged to consider the child as embedded in a family, school, and community context. Within this guiding framework, changes can promote individual social competency and create environments that foster and support the continued growth of social skills. If we are to expect inclusion to be a successful practice, it is necessary to develop systems that facilitate positive inclusion opportunities and value the learning experience it provides.

This task is multifaceted. First, children with autism must be supported to develop adequate communicative skills to function at a level that allows them to interact with their peers. Once these skills are developed, they must then be fostered in ways that improve social interactions. Through targeted interventions, addressing the core deficits of autism throughout the developmental trajectory, children can acquire skills and the social competences necessary for positive interactions with their families and peers. Given the variability of autism spectrum disorders, interventions must be tailored to address all domains that affect social communication and functioning and also deliver specific support, contingent on the child's social profile. Targeted interventions, addressing different developmental periods throughout the life course, can be an effective way to improve outcomes and provide meaningful skills and opportunities for social engagement in school and life contexts.

References

American Psychological Association. (2000). *Diagnostic and statistical manual of mental disorders* (4th ed.). Washington, DC: APA.

Baron-Cohen, S., Tager-Flusberg, H., & Cohen, D. (1994). *Understanding other minds: Perspectives from autism.* London, UK: Oxford University.

Barry, T., Klinger, L., Lee, J., Palardy, N., Gilmore, T., & Bodin Douglas, S. (2002). Examining the effectiveness of an outpatient clinic-based social skills group for high-functioning children with autism. *Journal of Autism and Developmental Disorders, 33*(6), 685-701.

Bauminger, N. (2002). The facilitation of social-emotional understanding and social interaction in high-functioning children with autism: Intervention outcomes. *Journal of Autism and Developmental Disorders, 32*(4), 283-298.

Bellini, S., Peters, J. K., Benner, L., & Hopf, A. (2007). A meta-analysis of school-based social skills interventions for children with autism spectrum disorders. *Remedial and Special Education, 28*(3), 153-162.

Buhrmester, D. (1990). Intimacy of friendship, interpersonal competence, and adjustment during preadolescence and adolescence. *Child Development, 61*(4), 1101-1111.

Burack, J., Root, R., & Zigler, E. (1997). Inclusive education for students with autism: Reviewing ideological, empirical, and community considerations. In D. J. Cohen & F. R. Volkmar (Eds.), *Handbook of autism and pervasive developmental disorders* (pp. 796-807). New York, NY: Wiley.

Capps, L., Sigman, M., & Yirmiya, N. (1996). Self-competence and emotional understanding in high-functioning children with autism. *Development and Psychopathology, 7,* 137-149.

Carr, E. G., & Darcy, M. (1990). Setting generality of peer modeling in children with autism. *Journal of Autism and Developmental Disorders, 20*(1), 45-59.

Education for All Handicapped Children Act of 1975, 20 U.S.C. § 612(5)(B).

Erikson, E. H. (1968). *Identity, youth and crisis.* New York, NY: Norton.

Gresham, F. (1986). Strategies for enhancing the social outcomes of mainstreaming: A necessary ingredient for success. In C. Meisel, *Mainstreaming handicapped children: Outcomes, controversies, and new directions* (pp. 193-218). Hillsdale, NJ: Erlbaum.

Guralnick, M. J. (1990). Social competence and early intervention. *Journal of Early Intervention, 14*(1), 3-14.

Gutstein, S., & Whitney, T. (2002). Asperger syndrome and the development of social competence. *Focus on Autism and Other Developmental Disabilities, 17*(3), 161-171.

Hobson, P. (2002).*The cradle of thought: Exploring the origins of thinking.* London: Macmillan.

Howlin, P., Goode, S., Hutton, J., & Rutter, M. (2004). Adult outcome for children with autism. *Journal of Child Psychology and Psychiatry, 45*(2), 212-229.

Individuals with Disabilities Education Act Amendments of 1997, 2004, 20 U.S.C. § 1400 *et seq.*

Kanner, L. (1943). Autistic disturbances of affective contact. *Nervous Child, 2,* 217-250.

Kasari, C., Locke, J., Gulsrud, A., & Rotheram-Fuller, E. (2011). Social networks and friendships at school: Comparing children with and without ASD. *Journal of Autism and Developmental Disorders, 41,* 533-544.

Kasari, C., Gulsrud, A., Wong, C., Kwon, S., & Locke, J. (2010). Randomized controlled caregiver mediated joint engagement intervention for toddlers with autism. *Journal of Autism and Developmental Disorders,40*(9),1045-1056.

Kasari, C., Paparella, T., Freeman, S., & Jahromi, L. (2008). Language outcome in autism: Randomized comparison of joint attention and play interventions. *Journal of Consulting and Clinical Psychology, 76*(1), 125-137.

Kasari, C., Freeman, S., & Paparella, T. (2006). Joint attention and symbolic play in young children with autism: A randomized controlled intervention study. *Journal of Child Psychology and Psychiatry, 47*(6), 611-620.

Kasari, C., Freeman, S., Bauminger, N., & Alkin, M. (1999). Parental perspectives on inclusion: Effects of autism and down syndrome. *Journal of Autism and Developmental Disorders, 29*(4), 297-305.

Laugeson, E., Frankel, F., Mogil, C., & Dillon, A. (2008). Parent-assisted social skills training to improve friendships in teens with autism spectrum disorders. *Journal of Autism and Developmental Disorders, 39*(4), 596-606.

Lawton, K., & Kasari, C. (2011). Brief report: Longitudinal improvements in the quality of joint attention in preschool children with autism. *Journal of Autism and Developmental Disorders, 42,* 307-312.

Lifter, K., Sulzer-Azaroff, B., Anderson, S., & Cowdery, G. E. (1993). Teaching play activities to preschool children with disabilities: The importance of developmental considerations. *Journal of Early Intervention, 17,* 139–159.

Locke, J., Ishijimia, E., Kasari, C., & London, N. (2010). Loneliness, friendship quality and the social networks of adolescents with high-functioning autism in an inclusive setting. *Journal of Research in Special Educational Needs, 10*(2), 74-81.

Lovaas, O.I. (1987). Behavioral treatment and normal educational and intellectual functioning in young autistic children. *Journal of Consulting and Clinical Psychology, 55,* 3-9.

McGee, G., Morrier, M., & Daily, T. (1999). An incidental teaching approach to early intervention for toddlers with autism. *Journal of the Association for Persons with Severe Handicaps, 24*(3), 133-146.

Miller, P., & Ingham, J. (1976). Friends, confidants, and symptoms. *Social Pyschiatry, 11,* 51-58.

Mundy, P., Hogan, A., & Doehring, P. (1996). *A preliminary manual for the abridged early social-communication scales (ESCS).* Coral Gables, FL: University of Miami. (Available from http://www.psy.miami.edu/ faculty/pmundy)

Mundy, P., Sigman, M., & Kasari, C. (1990). A longitudinal study of joint attention and language development in autistic children. *Journal of Autism & Developmental Disorders, 20,* 115-128.

No Child Left Behind (NCLB) Act of 2001, Pub. L. No. 107-110, § 115, Stat. 1425 (2002).

Ochs, E., Kremer-Sadlik, T., Solomon, O., & Sirota, K. G. (2001). Inclusion as social practice: Views of children with autism. *Social Development, 10*(3), 399-419.

Orsmond, G. I., Krauss, M. W., & Seltzer, M. M. (2004). Peer relationships and social and recreational activities among adolescents and adults with autism. *Journal of Autism and Developmental Disorders, 34,* 245–56.

Pierce-Jordan, S., & Lifter, K. (2005). Interaction of social and play behaviors in preschoolers with and without pervasive developmental disorder. *Topics in Early Childhood Special Education, 25*(1) 34-47.

Rocha, M. L., Schreibman, L., & Stahmer, A. C. (2007). Effectiveness of training parents to teach joint attention in children with autism. *Journal of Early Intervention, 29,* 154–172.

Rogers, S. J. (2000). Interventions that facilitate socialization in children with autism. *Journal of Autism and Developmental Disorders. Special Issue: Treatments for People with Autism and Other Pervasive Developmental Disorders: Research Perspectives, 30*(5), 399-409.

Sale, P., & Carey, D. (1995). The sociometric status of students with disabilities in a full-inclusion school. *Exceptional Children, 62,* 6-19.

Sigman, M., & Ruskin, E. (1999). Continuity anad change in the social competence of children with autism, Down syndrome, and developmental delays. *Monographs of the Society for Research in Child Development, 64,* 114.

Villa, R. A., Thousand, J. S., & Rosenberg, R. L. (1995). Creating heterogeneous schools: A systems change perspective. *Journal of Autism and Developmental Disorders, 37,* 1858-1868.

Wing, L., & Gould, J. (1979). Severe impairments of social interaction and associated abnormalities in children: Epidemiology and classification. *Journal of Autism and Developmental Disorders, 9*(1), 11-29.

6

Social Competence:
What It Is, Why It Is Important, and How PRT Can Achieve It
Daniel Openden

Joseph simply didn't take the skills he learned in Discrete Trial Training to any other contexts in his life. His parents were terribly frustrated. What good was it that he said hello to his teacher in the cubby when given the instruction, "Say hi," if he ignored his grandparents when they rang the doorbell? How useful was it that he could take turns in putting pennies in a jar when seated at a table with his teacher if he cut the line on the slide at the playground and grabbed the dice with his siblings?

While Sarah had learned to do what her teachers did on request (touch nose, clap hands), it was about as unmotivating as you can imagine. She hated it, did it just to get out of the chair, and never seemed at all interested. Most unnerving, she NEVER imitated anyone outside of these sessions. So, her parents thought, "When will she really get the hang of imitation, do it spontaneously, do it without being asked to do it? Will it happen? Can it happen?"

Joseph and Sarah's parents are struggling with social skill development. What is the real purpose of social skill training? How can children with autism be taught so that real world changes happen? How can the way we teach matter to them, motivate them, help establish a connection with them?

These are examples of the questions and struggles that motivate instructors in Pivotal Response Training. We want to focus on the conditions that are the most motivating, which have the highest chance of teaching skills that matter, that will occur spontaneously, and that will transfer across settings and people.

What Is Social Competence?

The social deficits of individuals with autism spectrum disorders are well known and well documented. There is a great deal of clarity and consensus on what constitutes social deficiency. Clinicians and researchers are much less clear and in much less agreement on social competence, but it has received a great deal of attention in recent years.

Social competence is an evolving concept that is broadly defined in the literature (Spence, 2003). Generally, social competence refers to the integration of social, emotional, and cognitive skills and behaviors that individuals need for successful engagement and interaction. The skills and behaviors expected vary with the age of the individual, cultural expectations, and the demands of a particular social situation. Social competence is not comprised of distinct skills; rather, it is defined by the abilities to receive social information, interpret social cues, and adjust behavior to the social expectations of the circumstance.

Why focus on a concept such as social competence? Socially competent individuals may have an easier time navigating the social world, developing meaningful friendships, working collaboratively in group and team contexts, pleasing authority figures, and managing complex situations. They may also ultimately encounter greater success in getting and in maintaining a job. Essentially, an individual's social competence is likely to significantly influence his or her quality of life, level of reinforcement, and personal happiness.

How successful have we been in achieving social competence in individuals with autism? This is difficult to evaluate, as most explorations have not even considered social skills in such a broad context. The literature has focused mainly on teaching children with autism spectrum disorders social skills as individual target behaviors. The general assumption that underlies this method is that the more skills you have, the more socially competent you are likely to be. However, a meta-analysis of social skills interventions by Bellini, Peters, Benner, & Hopf (2007) indicated that results are mixed and many commonly used interventions are not effective.

Many social skills programs emphasize teaching social "rules" that focus on what to do in a given context. While this can be a very effective teaching strategy that results in the ability to perform a given social skill under specific conditions, generalization of the skill is often lacking, particularly in natural settings. It is a clinical conundrum: how do we help prepare learners for the myriad situations they are likely to encounter and still teach efficiently? It is simply impossible to teach and prepare learners for *every* circumstance they may face. An alternative and more efficient model is needed.

Pivotal Response Treatment

Pivotal Response Treatment (PRT) is a naturalistic behavioral approach for children with ASDs (Koegel & Koegel, 2006; National Research Council, 2001) that may be particularly useful for improving broadly defined social competence. PRT is based on the science of applied behavior analysis (ABA). However, PRT does not primarily focus on the improvement of *individual* target behaviors, as traditional ABA approaches may have done. PRT targets *pivotal* areas that are aligned with the core symptoms of autism and teaches these pivotal behaviors in generalized ways. The major assumption of teaching via PRT is that when these core deficits are changed, generalized improvements occur across many behaviors.

To date, the literature has identified four pivotal areas for intervention: 1) motivation, 2) responsivity to multiple cues, 3) self-management, and 4) self-initiations (Koegel, Openden, Fredeen, & Koegel, 2006). It may be that social competence and PRT address broad areas for intervention in autism. A focus on pivotal areas in PRT may lead to improvements in, and the development of, social competence in individuals with ASD.

Over 20 years of empirical evidence support the efficacy and effectiveness of PRT for children with ASDs. PRT was first piloted and studied as the Natural Language Paradigm (NLP). NLP was designed to systematically include elements of natural language interactions into an ABA program. This was done to potentially improve the generalization and maintenance of treatment gains. In two critically important studies, the NLP demonstrated more rapid and generalized improvements in prompted, deferred, and spontaneous speech than in an analogue behavioral intervention (Koegel, Koegel, & Surratt, 1992; Koegel, O'Dell, & Koegel, 1987). Furthermore, in a critical review of eight published studies, Delprato (2001) indicated that naturalistic behavioral approaches were more effective at improving language compared to traditional discrete trial training (DTT) interventions.

Perhaps most intriguingly, Koegel, Koegel, & Surratt (1992) showed collateral decreases in problem behavior. This study represents the first PRT-based study that demonstrated generalized improvement in an untargeted behavior. As more studies began showing this effect, the NLP became Pivotal Response Treatment to more directly reference the broader targets and effects of the intervention. In essence, NLP evolved into PRT. The elements of NLP were preserved, and the intervention was extended into addressing core areas of deficit in individuals with autism.

A number of researchers have demonstrated that PRT was indeed an efficacious approach for increasing many different skills. Most importantly, documented changes in affect, play skills, and socialization have occurred with this intervention.

Several recent reviews and reports have also identified PRT as an evidence-based practice. In the report of the National Research Council (2001) that reviewed the most current research to date for educating young children with autism, PRT was included among the list of comprehensive programs. Simpson (2005) and Simpson et al. (2005) reviewed over 30 treatments for ASDs and categorized them into one of four categories: scientifically-based practice, promising practice, limited supporting information for practice, and not recommended. PRT was one of four interventions identified as a scientifically-based practice. In the same vein, the National Autism Center National Standards Report (2009) endeavored to give "comprehensive information about the level of scientific evidence that exists in support of the many educational and behavioral treatments currently available." PRT was identified as one of eleven established treatments. This is important to note, because many interventions purporting to address social skills do not have data that support their effectiveness. PRT is distinct because it does.

The efficacy and effectiveness of PRT are clear, but it is not clear what the relationship is between PRT and the development of social competence. In general, measures of social competence have not been employed in studies where PRT was implemented. In some ways, the field is still defining such concepts and methods for determining them.

Early Emergence of PRT from Traditional Discrete Trial Training

What Does It Look Like? All of the naturalistic strategies emerged from discrete trial training (DTT). PRT in particular emerged from other naturalistic approaches, most notably Natural Language Paradigm. In some ways, it is best understood in contrast to these traditional DTT teaching contexts. The NLP primarily focused on teaching language in a more naturalistic context that more closely resembled the way typically developing children learn to produce speech. The first goal of the NLP, then, was to bring responding under the control of natural environmental stimuli, allowing children to better interact with and learn from real world environments. That is, the goal was for children to respond to and interact with things in their environments—for example, for a hungry child to retrieve items from the refrigerator.

This was in part a reaction against the formality of DTT, in which skills were often taught in isolation and in artificial contexts. For example, a child may have been taught to go to the door, even when it was not time to exit. Typically developing children become socially competent adults through the shaping of social behaviors learned from an early age in the real world, much of which is language-based (Hart & Risley, 1989, 1992, 1995). The idea in NLP and in PRT is to capitalize on natural situations to teach skills in communication and socialization. In this way, the natural process that unfolds in typically developing children is mimicked. While children with ASDs can certainly be taught to use language in highly contrived environments, it is possible that the more social aspects of language and social communication may be missed

How Does It Generalize? A second goal of the NLP was to improve the generalization and maintenance of skills taught during intervention. Skills that do not transfer to natural contexts, to those not involved in instruction, or to novel environments are simply not useful. While data indicated that many children with ASDs made great progress within traditional DTT programs, some did not maintain skills over time, while others failed to generalize their skills across settings or people. Thus, the NLP shifted from arbitrary reinforcers used in traditional DTT programs to natural reinforcers that were directly and functionally related to the child's communication, producing better generalization and maintenance of treatment gains. For example, a child may be reinforced for requesting a car while playing with a car as opposed to saying "car" to get a token. These improvements, particularly those in generalizing newly learned skills, relate directly to social competence. Individuals who are better able to maintain, as well as generalize social communication skills across environments and with different people, tend to be more socially competent than those whose skills are limited to specific settings or with only particular individuals.

The idea is that communication should be meaningful, should make a difference in the life of the individual, and should give him skills to navigate his world in ways that matter to him. Having language becomes meaningful when children are able to use it to communicate within a social context (e.g., between parent and child, with teachers and peers). By moving away from arbitrary reinforcers that were not functional to the interaction in favor of natural reinforcers that were directly related to the child's interest and communicative response, the NLP emphasized the social function of language.

Core Intervention Components for Implementing PRT

Implementing PRT requires early intervention, intervention in natural environments, and parent training. In the PRT model, intervention begins as early as possible and during the earliest stages of brain development to maximize treatment outcomes.

While there are many skills for children with ASDs to be taught within an intervention program, subtle social behaviors are often the most difficult to teach. When children are engaged in meaningful intervention within social contexts from an early age, appropriate social behaviors may be learned more incidentally, and, as children get older, may not need to be taught directly. Developing social competence may be mostly about practice. The number of opportunities to teach, learn, shape, and reinforce appropriate social behavior increases dramatically if we use every natural moment to teach.

Second, as a naturalistic behavioral intervention, PRT is implemented primarily in home, school, and community settings, addressing generalization and maintenance concerns directly. Indeed, problems with generalization may have more to do with the teaching and the environments in which intervention is delivered than with the child.

Thus, PRT does not remove children with ASDs from the typical settings in which we ultimately want the behaviors we teach to occur. Rather, intervention is delivered and embedded within real world environments. If we want children with ASDs to grow up to become socially competent individuals, then we need to regularly expose them to natural environmental stimulation and implement intervention in social contexts so that social behaviors can be more easily learned, maintained, and generalized. Why was this less likely to occur in training? It does create challenges in training, data collection, and the design of instructional sessions. However, the potential benefits are enormous.

Finally, parent training is central to the PRT model, as parents are often considered primary intervention agents. Research has shown that parents can learn to effectively implement intervention for children with autism, and it makes sense to teach parents the skill set that works. As discussed, intervention typically begins early and in the child's natural environment (i.e., home) where children spend the majority of their time interacting with their parents. Because reciprocal, natural interactions between a caregiver and child greatly influence child development (Wetherby & Prizant, 2000), it is critical that parents not only are involved in the treatment of their children, but also learn to implement intervention procedures accurately and consistently.

Parent training also likely improves both the quantity and intensity of treatment, as intervention can be delivered throughout the child's waking hours and is not solely dependent on a highly quality therapist. Children with ASDs should be engaged in meaningful learning opportunities for as much of the day as possible. Logically, training parents to implement PRT increases the number of hours of intervention and the opportunities for learning. Additionally, embedding intervention during typical, everyday parent-child interactions across all environments (e.g., home, grocery store, park, restaurants) may further drive the development of social competence.

Implementing PRT within Social Skills Interventions

PRT has also been used as the primary intervention for directly teaching social skills to children with ASD. While PRT is generally implemented within the context of play-based interactions, particularly for young children, Stahmer (1999) and colleagues have used PRT to target appropriate play skills in children with ASDs, including:

- object play (e.g., with toys),
- symbolic play (e.g., dress-up activities), and
- sociodramatic play (acting out roles).

Play skills are critical for early language and social development and likely relate to the development of prosocial behaviors and social competence.

One interesting extension of PRT that has promise is the use of peer-implemented interventions in which typically developing peers learn to use PRT with children with ASDs. Pierce and Schreibman (1995) taught typical peers to implement PRT strategies in the classroom and found that children with autism interacted for longer periods, initiated more, and paid better attention in social contexts.

Baker, Koegel, and Koegel (1998) utilized the obsessive interests of children with autism as the motivational variable for improving social interaction with peers on the playground. For instance, typical peers were taught to play a tag game on a giant outline of the United States for a child who had an intense interest in maps. Dramatic increases in social interactions were found and maintained during follow up. Perhaps more importantly, the children with autism in the study generalized social interactions during other play activities with peers. In a related study implemented with siblings, similar results were demonstrated when incorporating the thematic ritualistic activities of children with autism into typical games (Baker, 2000).

These kinds of novel interventions make a tremendous difference in the extent to which a child with ASD can be integrated into a classroom environment. Instead of trying to motivate the child with ASD to engage in non-preferred tasks, the typically developing peers were simply brought into a context that the child with ASD would enjoy. This type of thinking outside of traditional contexts characterizes the more naturalistic instructional approaches.

More recent studies have used cooperative arrangements to provide training in PRT for both typical peers and children with ASDs. Cooperative arrangements focus on mutually reinforcing activities to ensure that peers also receive reinforcement and maintain interactions with children with ASDs. Since social interaction occurs between people, it is really important to also look at how happy the siblings or classmates are when they are interacting with the child with ASD. If we seek more natural initiations and interactions, we must teach in situations that are pleasant and interesting for the play partners as well.

As a pivotal area, self-management has also demonstrated improvements in social behaviors, including generalized changes in untargeted social behaviors. Boettcher (2004) used self-management to teach socially appropriate conversation skills—skills that are often overlooked, yet essential for developing social competence. While children with ASDs have been taught to respond with on-topic comments, many do not initiate questions during social conversation. For instance, during baseline, when Boettcher presented one participant with a leading statement such as, "I saw a great movie last night," the child frequently directed the conversation back to his perseverative interest and responded, "Do you like elevators?" instead of asking about the movie. The children were subsequently taught to ask appropriate, on-topic questions that were related to the other person's interests (e.g., "What movie did you see?" or "Who did you go to the movies with?"), and they were taught to monitor the extent to which they did this. Data indicated that self-management was an efficacious intervention for teaching these social conversation skills and that the skills were maintained and generalized to new settings with new conversation partners (e.g., untrained adults or typically developing peers).

Collateral Improvements in Untargeted Social Behaviors

While increases in targeted social communication and social skills are critical for children with ASDs, collateral improvements in untargeted social behaviors may be the most important in the development of social competence. When focusing on pivotal areas of responding, these behaviors are not taught directly. The assumption, rather, is that they are generalized behaviors that emerge naturally as a result of the intervention. Consistent with this, many of the studies demonstrating efficacy of PRT have documented improvements in both targeted and untargeted behaviors (Koegel, Openden, Fredeen, & Koegel, 2006).

Perhaps of greatest social significance, there have been clear indications that affect (of both children and caregivers) improves. In other words, children treated with PRT generally appear happier on observation. In addition, parents taught to implement PRT generally appear to be less stressed, more natural, and more confident in their interactions with their children.

In fact, collateral improvements in positive affect—a measure of happiness, interest, and enthusiasm—that occur while PRT is implemented have been demonstrated across a number of studies. Schreibman, Kaneko, & Koegel (1991) compared the affect of parents who were trained in PRT versus those who were trained in a different behavioral intervention. Results indicated that parents in the PRT condition exhibited significantly more positive affect, suggesting that natural parent-child interactions may be easier and more effective. Significant differences were also found in a similar study that compared affect during family interactions at dinnertime (Koegel, Bimbela, & Schreibman, 1996). Why does this matter? If parents appear happier while interacting with their child, they may engage their child more often, creating opportunities for learning even during activities that would not typically be thought of as therapy time (e.g., dinnertime).

Improvements in child affect have been demonstrated with young children. Brookman-Frazee (2004) taught parents to implement PRT with their children. Decreased parent stress and increased parent confidence were observed, as well as improvements in child affect. Koegel, Vernon, and Koegel (2009) found that embedded social reinforcers such as praise produced collateral improvements in child-initiated social engagement across different kinds of interactions. Improvements in child affect likely indicate that the children in these studies were also enjoying these interactions. It may be that children who are enjoying interaction would also be less avoidant of, and more likely to engage in, social interactions. It seems logical that this pattern would be associated with increased social competence.

Most importantly, collateral improvements in positive affect in children with ASDs suggest that they may indeed be enjoying their interactions with others. Koegel and Frea (1993) used the pivotal area of self-management for targeting social communication skills in two adolescent boys with autism and found generalized improvements in facial expression and affect. This is an excellent finding; it is imperative that our interventions result in real-life improvements that make a difference in the lives of the individuals. Koegel, Werner, Vismara, and Koegel (2005) used PRT during play dates to improve reciprocal social interactions and also found improvements in positive affect for the children with autism and their typically developing peers. Again, if we look at global social outcomes, this is a significant finding. The consumers of services include the parents, classmates, and friends of individuals with autism.

While there are extensive data that support the efficacy of the model, PRT does not appear to be implemented as widely as other approaches. With the continuing rise in the incidence of autism spectrum disorders in the United States to 1:10 (Centers for Disease, Control, and Prevention, 2009), the need to translate efficacious interventions into effective and accessible practice is urgent. In addition to the publication of training manuals (Koegel, Koegel, Bruinsma, Brookman, & Fredeen, 2003; Koegel, Schreibman, Good, Cerniglia, Murphy, & Koegel, 1989) and a book that covers communication,

social, and academic development (Koegel & Koegel, 2006), translational research studies have demonstrated the effective dissemination of PRT. There
is a gap between what is known to be effective and what is actually implemented. More children need access to interventions that have been demonstrated to be effective.

In addition, the number of children reached could be substantially increased if highly trained professionals spent less time working directly with
children and more time training parents to implement intervention. This is
one of the most important potential advantages to PRT. Symon (2005) assessed the spread of effect of parent training by asking parents to train other
significant caregivers in PRT (e.g., spouse, grandparent) once they returned
home. Parents were able to successfully train others, and the children made
gains in communication and behavior with other caregivers. Thus, parents
can not only learn to implement PRT correctly, but also train others who regularly interact with their child, further expanding the number of individuals
who receive effective services and increasing the number of hours in which
effective intervention is available for any individual child.

References

American Psychiatric Association. (1994). *Diagnostic and statistical manual for mental disorders* (4th ed.). Washington, DC: American Psychiatric Press.

Baker, M. J. (2000). Incorporating the thematic ritualistic behaviors of children with autism into games. *Journal of Positive Behavior Interventions, 2,* 66-84.

Bellini, S., Peters, J. K., Benner, L., & Hopf, A. (2007). A meta-analysis of school-based social skills interventions for children with autism spectrum disorders. *Remedial and Special Education, 28,* 153-162.

Boettcher, M. A. (2004). Teaching social conversation skills to children with autism through self-management: An analysis of treatment gains and meaningful outcomes. (Unpublished doctoral dissertation).

Brookman-Frazee, L. (2004). Using parent/clinician partnerships in parent education programs for children with autism. *Journal of Positive Behavior Interventions, 6,* 195-213.

Centers for Disease Control and Prevention. (2009). Prevalence of autism spectrum disorders: Autism and developmental disabilities monitoring network, United States 2006. *Morbidity and Mortality Weekly Report 2009, 58,* 1-24.

Delprato, D. J. (2001). Comparisons of discrete-trial and normalized behavioral language intervention for young children with autism. *Journal of Autism and Developmental Disorders, 31,* 315-325.

Hart, B., & Risley, T. R. (1989). The longitudinal study of interactive systems. *Education and Treatment of Children, 12,* 347-358.

Hart, B., & Risley, T. R. (1992). American parenting of language-learning children: Persisting differences in family-child interactions observed in natural home environments. *Developmental Psychology, 28,* 1096-1105.

Hart, B., & Risley, T. R. (1995). Meaningful differences in the everyday experiences of young American children. Baltimore: Paul H. Brookes.

Koegel, L. K., Camarata, S. M., Valdez-Manchaca, M., & Koegel, R. L. (1998). Setting generalization of question-asking by children with autism. *American Journal on Mental Retardation, 102,* 346-357.

Koegel, R. L., Bimbela, A., & Schreibman, L. (1996). Collateral effects of parent training on family interactions. *Journal of Autism and Developmental Disorders, 26,* 347-359.

Koegel, R. L., & Frea, W. D. (1993). Treatment of social behavior in autism through the modification of pivotal social skills. *Journal of Applied Behavior Analysis, 26,* 369–377.

Koegel, R. L., Koegel, L. K., Bruinsma, Y., Brookman, L., & Fredeen, R. M. (2003). *Teaching first words to children with autism and communication delays using Pivotal Response Training.* Santa Barbara: University of California.

Koegel, R. L., Koegel, L. K., & Surratt, A. (1992). Language intervention and disruptive behavior in preschool children with autism. *Journal of Autism and Developmental Disorders, 22,* 141-153.

Koegel, R. L., Koegel, L. K., Vernon, T., and Brookman-Frazee, L. (2010). Empirically supported pivotal response treatment for children with autism spectrum disorders. In J.R. Weisz, & A. E. Kazdin, *Evidence-based psychotherapies for children and adolescents* (pp. 327-344). New York, NY: Guilford Press.

Koegel, R. L., O'Dell, M. C., & Koegel, L. K. (1987). A natural language teaching paradigm for nonverbal autistic children. *Journal of Autism and Developmental Disorders, 17,* 187-199.

Koegel, R. L., Openden, D., Fredeen, R. M., & Koegel, L. K. (2006). The basics of pivotal response treatment. In R. L. Koegel & L. K. Koegel (Eds.), *Pivotal Response Treatments for autism: Communication, social and academic development* (pp. 3-30). Baltimore: Paul H. Brookes.

Koegel, R. L., Schreibman, L., Good, A., Cerniglia, L., Murphy, C., & Koegel, L. K. (1989). *How to teach pivotal behaviors to children with autism: A training manual.* Santa Barbara: University of California.

Koegel, R. L., Werner, G. A., Vismara, L. A., & Koegel, L. K. (2005). The effectiveness of contextually supported play date interactions between children with autism and typically developing peers. *Research and Practice for Persons with Severe Disabilities, 30,* 93-102.

National Autism Center. (2009). *National standards report.* Randolph, MA: Author.

National Research Council. (2001). *Educating children with sutism.* Washington, DC: National Academy Press.

Openden, D. (2005). Pivotal Response Treatment for multiple families of children with autism: Effects of a 4-day group parent education workshop (Unpublished doctoral dissertation).

Pierce K., & Schreibman L. (1995). Increasing complex social behaviors in children with autism: Effects of peer-implemented pivotal response training. *Journal of Applied Behavior Analysis, 28,* 285–295.

Schreibman, L., Kaneko, W. M., & Koegel, R. L. (1991). Positive affect of parents of autistic children: A comparison across two teaching techniques. *Behavior Therapy, 22,* 479-490.

Simpson, R. L. (2005). Evidence-based practices for students with autism spectrum disorders. *Focus on Autism and Other Developmental Disorders, 20,* 140–149.

Simpson, R. L., de Boer-Ott, S. R., Griswold, D. E., Myles, B. S., Byrd, S. E., Ganz, J. B., et al. (2005). *Autism spectrum disorders: Interventions and treatments for children and youth.* Thousand Oaks, CA: Corwin Press.

Spence, S. H. (2003). Social skills training with children and young people: Theory, evidence, and practice. *Child & Adolescent Mental Health, 8,* 84-96.

Stahmer, A. C. (1999). Using Pivotal Response Training to facilitate appropriate play in children with autistic spectrum disorders. *Child Language Teaching and Therapy, 15,* 29-40.

Symon, J. B. (2005). Expanding interventions for children with autism: Parents as trainers. *Journal of Positive Behavior Interventions, 7,* 159-173.

Wetherby, A., & Prizant, B. M. (2000). *Autism spectrum disorders: A transactional developmental perspective.* Baltimore: Paul H. Brookes.

7

Key Components of Social Skills Training

Jed Baker

Social skill challenges are a core feature of autism. Yet there is not widespread agreement about what social skills are, how to assess or measure them, or how best to teach them. In this chapter, I will lay out a working definition of social skills, discuss how to assess and measure them, and describe a flexible model to teach and generalize skills.

Definitional Issues: What Are Social Skills?

In the past, other authors have defined social skills as "interpersonal responses . . . that allow the child to adapt to the environment through verbal or non-verbal communication" (Mateson and Mateson, 2007) or "socially acceptable learned behaviors that enable a person to interact with others in ways that elicit positive responses and assist in avoiding negative responses" (Bellini & Peters, 2008).

What both these definitions have in common is the description of a *social context* (i.e., that these behaviors happen with other people around), and that the behaviors are *desirable* (i.e., "adaptive," "elicit positive responses"). Perhaps more simply put,

> *Social skills are desirable behaviors that occur in a social context. By desirable, we mean that the behaviors allow individuals to get more positive than negative responses from others.*

How Does This Definition Differ from Communication Skills?

It is the social context that defines social skills. Communication that occurs in the presence of others has the potential for social impact. Requests, initiations, and responses to others' initiations are all social. On the other hand, communication that primarily occurs in isolation might be considered to be self-stimulation, as when a child repeats certain noises to entertain himself. If that self-stimulation occurs around others and leads to positive responses from others, such as laughter, it may then serve a social function. Thus, it is not the exact words, noises, or gestures that differentiate communication skills from social skills, but the social function (the impact on others) that determines whether it is a social skill. Skinner's analysis of verbal behavior helps us to focus on the function of verbal communication rather than on just the structure of language, thus differentiating communication that is social from that which does not serve a social function.

How Does This Definition Differ from Replacement and Self-Regulation Skills?

Sometimes, a child's ability to manage his frustration has important social consequences, and sometimes it does not. If a child is all alone while trying to complete a puzzle, his ability to manage frustration may not have any social consequences, and we can say his frustration management skills are not social in this moment. However, most of the time, a child's ability to handle frustration has very important social consequences. A child who cannot manage his frustration in class may have fewer peers to play with, while the child who can manage himself may have more friends. What makes a replacement skill a desirable social skill? When that behavior leads to the child getting more positive than negative responses from others. For example, a child who engages in tantrums to avoid doing schoolwork would, on the one hand, get something he wants (avoiding work), but he might have to endure punishments from his teacher as well. Asking for help might be a more desirable social skill since the child could then manage the difficult work without enduring punishments.

Measuring Social Skills

Bellini and Peters (2008) review some of the various ways in which social skills are measured through observations, interviews, and rating scales. They distinguish between measures of "social competence," defined as judgments of that child's social ability by those who know the child well (e.g., parents and teachers), versus "social skills," which reflect observations of specific behaviors in particular settings.

Gresham et al. (2001) classify these social measures into three categories: type I, II, and III. Type I measures refer to rating scales and interviews that measure social competence. The Social Skills Rating System (Gresham and Elliot, 1990) is one norm-referenced measure of social competence for ages 3-18 designed for a broad population of students (i.e., not just students with ASD). The Social Responsiveness Scale (Constantino, 2005) is a norm-referenced measure specifically designed for students with ASD.

These broad measures may not assess the specific identified skill goals of a particular student. To measure specific skill goals for a student, one can create an individualized rating scale in which key stakeholders rate the targeted student on each targeted skill. Although these are subjective judgments from parents and teachers, Bellini and Peters (2008) describe them as socially valid measures of competence exactly because they represent the way those closest to the child perceive the child. These measures reflect the specific community standards that are embedded in the perceptions of those judging the targeted student. Although these measures represent a summary of how that student might behave across settings, they may not be sensitive to small changes in behavior in specific settings.

Type II measures refer to observations of specific behaviors in particular settings. These more objective measures are very sensitive to changes in behavior, yet may be more challenging to collect across settings. Often these measures are criterion referenced. That is, a set of objective criteria are established to define accurate performance of a skill. The majority of single-case research designs in the behavioral literature (e.g., see Mateson and Mateson, 2007) have relied on direct observational measures.

Type III measures refer to role plays or discussions with the child to assess whether he knows how to perform a particular skill. For example, asking a child to tell or show you what he will do if he gets teased would be a type III measure. Because these assessments do not measure what the child will actually do in the natural environment, they are not as valid as, nor do they correlate with, type I and type II measures (Bellini and Peters, 2008).

Approaches to Teaching Skills

Some of the major approaches to skills training can be categorized based on their underlying assumptions of what leads to behavior change (see Table 1, pages 140-41). The behavioral approaches focus on altering observable events in the environment (antecedents and consequences) in order to increase certain behaviors and decrease undesirable behaviors. For example, an instructor might model and prompt a student to greet his peers and then reward the student for doing so. Cognitive behavioral approaches share some of these assumptions about manipulating the environment to change behavior, but they extend the notion to consider how an individual interprets or perceives what happens in the environment. To this end, individuals' thoughts and perceptions become a primary focus in understanding how someone will behave. For example, an instructor might explain to a student how others would think and feel if he did not greet his peers. Trying to alter the child's perceptions or interpretations of events can be accomplished with verbal explanation for high functioning youngsters, or through certain visual supports that make the abstract more concrete for youngsters with more language challenges.

Relationship-based approaches (e.g., Floortime and Son-Rise) posit that developing a trusting relationship is a primary factor in influencing the development of new skills. Through following the lead of the child, respecting his or her preferences, and sharing control of activities with the child, trust and motivation develop so that learning can occur.

Some of the approaches in Table 1 combine ideas from several categories. For example, some of the contemporary ABA approaches focus on shared control and respecting the child's preferences, a core value of the relationship-based approaches.

Table 1

Applied Behavioral Analysis-ABA: Focus on manipulating observable events (antecedents and consequences) to change behavior

ABA Approaches: Teaching skills usually involves cueing, modeling, and prompting appropriate behaviors, followed by reinforcing consequences for those positive behaviors. The older, traditional ABA approaches, like Discrete Trial Training (Lovaas, 1987), often occurred in one-on-one contrived settings and emphasized external reinforcers (food, access to other privileges, toys). Contemporary ABA approaches, like (Verbal Behavior Therapy) (VBT) (Sundberg and Partington, 1998) and Pivotal Response Treatment (PRT) (Koegel and Koegel, 2006), often occur in more natural settings and make efforts to increase intrinsic motivation to socialize by making the interaction fun in and of itself, rather than using a material reward after the interaction.

Video Modeling and Video Self-modeling: Bellini, Akullian, & Hopf, (2007), and Bellini & Akullian (2007) have shown that video can be used to show children how to engage with others, increase positive behaviors, and decrease disruptive behaviors.

Augmentative Communication and Visual Supports used in the Context of ABA: PECS system (Frost & Bondy, 2006) is one example in which pictures are used to help learners communicate their wants, replace negative behaviors, and eventually comment on their experiences as well.

Cognitive-Behavioral: Focus on expanding perspective taking along with manipulating observable events to change behavior	Relationship Based: Focus on creating engaging interactions, following the child's lead, in order to increase relatedness to others
Relationship Development Intervention (RDI): focuses on "Dynamic intelligence," which means being able to think flexibly, take different perspectives, cope with change, and process several sources of information simultaneously (Gutstein, 2007). **Social Thinking Model:** Garcia-Winner (2007) described a model of social development in which social thinking is required before the development of social skills. Social thinking involves the ability to take another's perspective to understand their intentions, thoughts, and feelings. From this knowledge comes the ability to interact with others effectively. **Social Stories:** Gray (1991) first described Social Stories as a way to help students understand social information about a particular situation. The stories are designed to explain social cues and other's perspectives in a particular situation to prepare a child to deal with that situation. **Structured Learning:** as described by Goldstein and his colleagues (McGuiness and Goldstein, 1997), involves four steps: modeling, role playing, social reinforcement, and transfer training (practice in natural settings). The modeling portion usually involves explanation of others' perceptions and social consequences of one's actions. Structured learning is a key component of the approach taken in several social skill manuals for individuals with autism spectrum disorders (Baker, 2003; 2005). **Visual Supports to Expand Understanding of Events and Tasks:** The TEACCH approach pioneered the use of many visual supports to make the sequence of daily activities predictable and tasks more understandable (Mesibov et al., 2005). Other examples include picture books (Baker, 2001; 2006) and closely related "First-Then" visual displays of activities to help individuals understand rewarding consequences for completing a task.	The objectives of **DIR®/ Floortime™** are to build "fundamental developmental capacities" for social, emotional, and intellectual growth, rather than focus on isolated behaviors. Floortime is both a technique, in which a caregiver gets down on the floor to interact with the child for twenty or more minutes at a time, and a philosophy that characterizes all daily interactions with the child. It involves following the lead of the child to gain motivation and trust and challenging the child to interact. **Son-Rise Program:** In 1976, Barry Kaufman first described the Son-Rise approach that he had used to successfully treat his son, Raun, who was severely autistic. The approach entails others joining the child in his/her world by mimicking his/her activities (Kaufman, 1994). The goal is to make people more attractive to the child than objects and obsessions. There is no direct research evaluating this method at this time.

What Evidence Is There for Various Teaching Approaches?

Deciding whether social skills training works is incredibly challenging, as the definition of social skills, the social skills targeted, and the ways to teach, generalize, and measure progress differ across studies. That being said, there is evidence that many of the strategies described in Table 1 can lead to positive changes using the types of measures described previously (i.e., type I, II, and III measures).

- Many of the ABA strategies, involving modeling, prompting, and reinforcement, have been shown to be effective in teaching a variety of social skills, including attention/eye contact, appropriate content and initiation of conversation, play skills, and frequency and duration of interactions (see Mateson and Mateson, 2007, for a review of 79 studies).
- Strategies that involve showing children what to do through video modeling and social stories have also shown positive results.
- Garcia-Winner's social thinking strategies are beginning to be investigated with the ASD population with some positive feedback.
- Structured learning enjoys a large evidence base with varied populations not specific to autism. Trimarchi (2004) investigated the use of the structured learning approach for those with Asperger syndrome using my social skills training manual (Baker, 2003) and found parents reported at least minimal improvement on 90 percent of targeted skills compared to a control group.
- RDI and DIR have also been shown to lead to positive changes in behavior, yet there is a lack of controlled studies evaluating these models—so we know many children improve, but we cannot always attribute that to the intervention.

A recent controlled study evaluated the effects of The Early Start Denver Model (ESDM), an early intervention program for children as young as 12 months old (see Dawson et al., 2009). Although the purpose of this study was not simply to evaluate social skills, such skills were certainly part of the outcome measures. This was a particularly interesting study because of the powerful results and the authors' emphasis on integrating aspects of applied behavioral analysis (ABA), particularly PRT strategies, with developmental and relationship-based approaches. In many ways, their emphasis on clearly defined skills training within a play-based approach truly represents the direction of contemporary ABA approaches as they blend with the values of relationship-based approaches that stress shared control between adult and child, and utilizing the preferences of the child to insure a positive experience. The study compared ESDM to a comparison group in which parents received recommendations on ASD interventions, as well as referrals to local community providers of the interventions. In the first year, children in the ESDM group gained 15.4 IQ points on average, while children in the comparison group gained an average of 4.4 points. Over the two-year study period, children in the ESDM group consistently improved on measures of communication skills, motor skills, and daily living skills compared to the control group.

Despite all these promising outcomes, there is still a gap between the science and practice of skills training in school settings. Back in 2007, Bellini, Peters, Benner, and Hopf challenged the social skills world after concluding that most school-based social skills training efforts were minimally effective according to their review of 55 outcome studies. These researchers pointed out the **problems with many school-based social skill interventions,** including:

- failure to match targeted goals to the child's needs,
- lack of generalization of skills into natural settings,
- short duration of treatment, and
- failure to motivate skill performance.

Each of these issues is discussed below.

Matching Strategy and Goals to Skill Needs

Bellini et al. (2007) and Mateson and Mateson (2007) point out that very few studies provide a rationale for selecting certain skill goals. Often schools provide a one-size-fits-all curriculum of skills to students without identifying whether the skill goals are relevant to the participating students. We must target skills that are relevant to the needs of the students, considering what skills are necessary for them to function successfully in particular settings. Bellini et al. (2007) also argue that we must distinguish between assessing the knowledge of a skill versus the ability to perform that skill in natural settings. This last issue relates to the next challenge, generalization.

Generalization

If interventions take place primarily in contrived, restricted settings, such as pullout therapy sessions, there is less likely to be generalization into the natural environment. Bellini et al. (2007) pointed to slightly better results for skills training that occurred in the classroom rather than in pullout sessions. Although it can be useful to begin skills training in structured, contrived settings, eventually skills will need to be prompted in the settings in which we want the skills to be enacted.

Duration or Dosage of Treatment

Gresham et al. (2001) concluded that skills training that lasts about 30 hours spread over 10 to 12 weeks is often not enough to see positive results. Bellini et al. (2007) used this conclusion to suggest that 30 hours spread over 10 to 12 weeks ought to be the minimum when providing social skills training.

Motivation

Bellini et al. (2007) discussed the issue of motivation as it relates to the performance of previously learned skills. Although a child may *know* what to do, lack of reinforcement may make it difficult to *perform* skills when needed, which may in part account for the mediocre effects seen in school-based skills training studies.

Putting It All Together: Key Components of Effective Social Skills Training

Based on the outcome research described above, there are certain critical components of skills training that must be considered in order to ensure skills are taught effectively. I have outlined a flexible model to address many of these components (Baker, 2003; 2005). The goal of the model is to improve the quality of life for children and their families by increasing students' ability to negotiate social situations effectively, cope with frustrations, reduce negative behaviors, and develop friendships. The model involves the following five key components:

1. **Assessment:** Prioritize relevant skill goals based on input from key stakeholders (e.g., the student, parents, and teachers).
2. **Motivation:** Establish motivation to learn and use skills across settings.
3. **Skill acquisition:** Teach skills using strategies that match the student's language, cognitive, and attention abilities.
4. **Generalization:** Coach students to use the skills in natural settings and involve those who surround the targeted student.
5. **Peer sensitivity:** Train typical peers as necessary to increase generalization of skills with peers, reduce isolation, increase opportunities for friendship, and decrease bullying.

Each component is explained briefly below.

Assessment of Social Skills

Assessment involves three related issues: 1) How do we determine relevant skill goals to target? 2) In what order should we teach skills—is there a particular sequence? 3) How can we measure initial status and progress toward skill goals?

It would simplify the assessment process if there were one core set of skills from which to evaluate the functioning of any particular individual. However, given our definition of social skills (i.e., behaviors that are desirable in a social context), it is likely that desirable behaviors vary across social settings. As a result, the local social context must be taken into account when considering what skills to target.

As described earlier, recent reviews of social skills training in school-based programs suggest that trying to teach a universal set of skills in a short amount of time (e.g., 10-12 weeks) has not been effective. Instead, it has been suggested that we focus on specific, relevant skill deficits of a student and work on them for a longer period of time. I ask that students, caring professionals, and family members surrounding the student help prioritize three to four skills to work on for months at a time across settings. There is nothing magical about the number three or four, yet this is a manageable number of skill goals if we are going to require parents and teachers to consistently prompt these skills to ensure generalization across settings.

Identifying Socially Relevant Goals

In order to assess the needs within a particular social context, I take a client-centered approach that involves assessing the specific wishes and concerns of the client and key caretakers surrounding that individual. Key players typically include the individual with autism, parents, teachers, and employers. We ask them to identify the settings in which they hope that child will function successfully. We then ask two simple questions about those settings in order to target skills:

1. What does this individual do too much of in that setting that may interfere with the ability to function? Excess behaviors might include becoming aggressive when confronted with difficult work, becoming aggressive when denied a desired item or activity, touching others, interrupting, talking endlessly about one's own interests, or insulting others. This information leads to the identification of "replacement skills" (i.e., more adaptive behaviors that allow the individual to get what he or she needs without bothering others).

2. What does that individual not do enough of in order to function in that setting? These behavioral deficits often include attending skills, initiation skills, responding to others, asking for help, asserting one's wishes or needs.

We ask the key players to agree on three or four skills we should prioritize as targets to begin treatment. As children master skills, we can target new skills, but to begin, it is best to keep the initial targets at a manageable number.

As key players try to identify skills relevant for the desired settings, we offer them a "menu" of skills from which to choose (see Baker, 2003; 2005). This menu is by no means exhaustive and is not meant to be a universal core set of skills. It does, however, provide these key players with the words to articulate some of the skills they might feel are relevant. They may choose, however, to articulate their own skill goal that is not identified on the menu but nonetheless relevant for functioning in an identified setting. Within this menu, there are certain categories of skills, including:

- Initiating and responding skills for play
- Initiating and responding skills for conversation
- Frustration management skills
- Conflict management skills

In some ways, these are clusters of skills and targeting one in a cluster may simplify learning others in that cluster.

Are There Sequences of Skills?

In deciding what skills to target, I do not subscribe to a model in which skills must be taught in a certain sequence. Instead, I take a functional approach in which I ask what skills are necessary for the student to function in a desired setting. That being said, there are two categories of skills that are prerequisites for many other skills: *joint attention* and *symbolic communication skills.*

Joint attention refers to the child's ability to attend to what the instructor (parent or teacher) is attending to. In other words, a child must attend in order to learn. Symbolic communication refers to the ability to communicate about events, objects, or people when those events, objects, or people are not concretely present to the child. An "intraverbal" (a Skinnerian term) refers to this ability to respond to a verbal question with verbal information independent of visual prompts. For example, if a child can respond to the question, "What did you have for breakfast?" describing what he ate without referring to pictures of the breakfast foods, then it suggests the child can "talk about" events or objects in the absence of those events. This kind of ability is a prerequisite for conversation about the past, future, or hypothetical situations. If a child is not able to do this, he will not easily be able to discuss situations or learn only from verbal explanation, which is a primary way many children are introduced to new topics in school. Without good symbolic language skills, children will need to see pictures or videos of events or actually be in the event in order to learn about it.

How Do We Measure Initial Status and Progress towards Goals?

In clinical practice, I rarely use norm-referenced measures, as they tend to provide too gross a picture of the student's social skills and not specific enough to measure the skills we may have targeted. To ensure we measure the specific skill goals for a student, I often create an individualized rating scale in which we have the key stakeholders rate the targeted student on a five-point Likert Scale for each targeted skill (see Figure 1). Although these are subjective judgments from parents and teachers, Bellini and Peters (2008) describe them as socially valid measures of competence because they represent the way those closest to the child perceive the child. Others' opinions of the child's behavior reflect local community standards for behavior and are thus socially valid measures.

When possible, I try to get type II measures (i.e., direct observations of behavior) as well. These measures are criterion referenced—that is, a set of objective criteria is established to define accurate performance of a skill so that it is possible to define when a skill has been mastered. To determine whether skills are generalizing over time and across settings, it is useful to keep track of when the behaviors occur prompted versus unprompted. Spontaneous performance of skills suggest the student can more independently use those skills even when key staff members are not available to prompt skill use.

In practice, it is certainly possible to get these observational measures of students when there are support staff members to take data. When a child does not have a dedicated aide to keep track of behaviors each day, a special education support staff member may come in periodically to take data at certain times during the week to sample behavior. However, it is often difficult to get these observational measures in mainstream classrooms with high functioning students who have little access to support staff to take data in a regular way. In contrast, I have found it exceedingly simple to get the individualized ratings (Figure 1) in typical school settings for all students. This is an important consideration in bridging the gap between science and practice. We must be able to measure social skill changes, yet we need to be aware of what is feasible in any given setting.

Figure 1

Skill Rating Form

Name_____

Parent/Teacher_____

<u>Directions</u>: Based on your observations, rate each student's use of the following skills according to the scale below:

1 = Student **never** uses the skill
2 = Student **rarely** uses the skill
3 = Student **sometimes** uses the skill
4 = Student **often** uses the skill
5 = Student **almost always** uses the skill

Skills	Dates			

Motivation

Just because we identify social skill goals does not mean a student is motivated to learn those skills. One of the key issues in working with students with autism is how to motivate a desire to socialize with others. Can a child who tends to avoid social contact learn to desire social interaction? Can social interaction itself be a reinforcer?

What Is a Social Reinforcer?

Any response that leads to an increase in behavior is considered a reinforcer. Social reinforcers would be social responses by others that lead to increases in behavior in the targeted student. In other words, social interaction itself becomes the reward. It is difficult to distinguish what is and is not a social reinforcer, given that any reaction by an adult (including providing food) could *theoretically* be defined as social since it occurs in a social context. The question becomes, "Does the child behave in order to interact with the adult (a socially motivated action) or in order to get a material reward (not necessarily social)?"

For many of us, getting material presents from loved ones has both material and social meaning. Without being able to get inside the individual's head, it is hard to know what the true function of the behavior is. In practice, the true function of the behavior is not always known and social reinforcers are typically defined by how they look, with praise, laughter, a smile, physical contact, and verbal and nonverbal communication being described as "social." Food, toys, and other material rewards are typically not considered social reinforcers, even though they may have a social function.

How Can Individuals Learn to Be Motivated by Social Reinforcement?

The debate over what leads to social motivation underscores two broad views of motivation: *extrinsic* and *intrinsic.*

One way social motivation is theorized to develop is by pairing *extrinsic rewards* with social interaction. For example, if we want a child to play a game with others, we might provide a desired food or toy after he plays the game with others. Such a reward is considered extrinsic to the activity because it is given after the game rather than built into the game. Over time, we might expect the social interaction to become motivating because it was historically associated with extrinsic rewards.

Another way to motivate social interaction is to attempt to make the interaction **intrinsically motivating.** Here we would attempt to make the social interaction itself more interesting by incorporating favored activities into the social interaction rather than afterwards. For example, if a child likes to wrap himself in a blanket, we could make a game of wrapping him in the blanket and pulling the blanket off, prompting the child to request being wrapped. Here the reward is built in, or intrinsic to, the social interaction.

Table 2 summarizes several ways to motivate students to learn and enact skills. The table is divided into those strategies that emphasize extrinsic motivation (i.e., rewards after skill use) and those that emphasize intrinsic motivation (i.e., making skill use itself rewarding). The table is also divided into those strategies useful for those students with fewer symbolic communication abilities who cannot talk about situations or events in the abstract, versus those with good symbolic communication skills who can discuss past and future events and other abstract concepts such as how people think and feel. For those with excellent symbolic communication, it is possible to "talk them into" wanting to learn skills by highlighting the positive consequences of skill use, such as the promise of extrinsic rewards and achievement of future goals. Those with fewer symbolic skills, and therefore less ability to maintain a future orientation, need more immediate extrinsic rewards or to experience intrinsic pleasure from the activities themselves.

In practice, I have found it crucial to maintain a flexible approach, utilizing both extrinsic and intrinsic strategies. I would prefer a child to be motivated to socialize because he or she "intrinsically" enjoys it. In order to establish this, I need to discover which activities will be enjoyable to the child, using his or her strengths and preferences as a guide. Yet sometimes a child's repertoire of preferred activities is extremely limited, and in order to "try out" a new activity, I need to initially use extrinsic rewards to motivate the child to try the new activity. After some experience with the new activity, the child may begin to enjoy it and thus develop intrinsic interest in the activity, no longer requiring a reward after the activity. In the last section of this chapter, I will describe the approach to build motivation taken with two very different students, one with limited symbolic language, and one with excellent symbolic language and intellectual skills.

Initial Skill Acquisition: Variants of Modeling and Prompting

For all students with autism spectrum disorders, I believe it is crucial to model and prompt skill use in natural settings. There is certainly a great deal of research to support these general strategies (Mateson and Mateson, 2007). This cannot be done as effectively without addressing the motivational issues described earlier. In other words, it makes no sense to continually prompt a child to initiate a game if he or she never enjoys the game. The child would

Table 2

	Extrinsic Rewards	Intrinsic Rewards
Pre-Symbolic Language	Use of material rewards such as food, toys, privileges, or social praise provided after skill enactment. The reward may have no natural connection to the skill in that the reward may not be available in naturally occurring settings. This characterized the earlier **Lovaas discrete trial** approach, yet the more contemporary Lovaas approach utilizes intrinsic approaches as well.	**Pivotal Response Training** often embeds the child's interests into the skill lesson, and intersperses challenging tasks with easier ones to maintain intrinsic motivation. **Verbal Behavior Training** starts with "mand" training in which the child learns to request favored items or activities, so that the skill lesson and the reward are naturally connected; the reward is intrinsic to the learning situation. **DIR®/Floortime**™ and the **Son-Rise Program** follow the child's lead to gain motivation. **RDI** attempts to make social referencing fun and engaging in and of itself
Good Symbolic Language	Extrinsic rewards are provided as above, yet often through the accumulation of symbolic rewards such as tokens or points on a behavior chart.	**Explain rationale** for working on challenging skills; that it will help the student reach his or her own future goals **For students who seem not to care** about their future, increase self-awareness of strengths and talents to establish future goals prior to focusing on their challenges **Have students teach** necessary skills to others to help them feel competent themselves **Make socializing fun** through high interest activities

only learn to repeat the words to ask to play and then drift away from actually playing the game. Only with proper motivation (intrinsic or extrinsic) can we model and prompt skill use.

There are two considerations in deciding how we will model and prompt skill use. First is the type of *strategy* used. This depends on the symbolic language and cognitive skills of the students. Those with good symbolic language can benefit from strategies in which skill steps are explained prior to being modeled and prompted. Many of the cognitive-behavioral strategies in Table 1 can be used with such students who are capable of understanding others' perspectives and subtle social cues when they are explained or highlighted for them. My preferred approach is to explain, model, and role-play skills (the structured learning approach) prior to prompting skill use in natural settings.

For students who have great deficits in symbolic language, we cannot "talk about" how to perform a skill. Rather, the instructor must show how to do the skill by modeling and prompting the student in the actual situation and perhaps supplement the student's understanding of what to do by showing pictures or video of the skill steps in the actual situation. Many of the ABA strategies in Table 1 do not require a high level of symbolic language. In addition, picture books (Baker, 2001, 2006) and video modeling (Bellini and Akullian, 2007) may also require less symbolic language, as they are visually based techniques.

The second issue to consider in skill acquisition is *where to teach* the skills: in groups, classrooms, or individually. There is evidence that teaching in a classroom can increase generalization, given that skills are learned in the place where they most need to be performed. There are, however, benefits to smaller group instruction in which students have a chance to befriend each other. Positive results were found for this type of group instruction provided in my social skills training manual. (See Trimarchi, 2004, for a controlled outcome study on group training described by Baker, 2003.) If students have significant behavioral challenges and difficulties attending in group settings, it may be best to begin with individual treatment prior to considering a group. This does not mean that we cannot try to generalize skills into a group setting, but the initial acquisition of skills may need to be conducted in a one-on-one setting where there are fewer distractions.

Generalization

In addition to establishing extrinsic or intrinsic motivation to perform skills as described above, students need reminders and coaching to perform skills in natural settings. In Bellini et al.'s (2007) review of skills training studies, coaching in natural situations was often a missing ingredient in social skills training efforts and one of the reasons for mediocre results. I have found it crucial to create written reminders (cue cards, behavior charts, or skill lesson sheets) for parents and teachers working with students. These written reminders are sent home to parents, and distributed to the child's teachers. Ideally, parents and teachers should have the opportunity to not only hear what they should prompt their students to do, but to actually observe how the student can be prompted. This kind of instruction to teachers and parents is typically lacking, yet perhaps a large contributor to the positive effects seen in programs such as The Early Start Denver Model.

I typically instruct parents and teachers to do three things to help students remember to perform skills: *Prime* students before situations in which they will need to use the skills, *coach* students during skill enactment, and *review* with students afterwards how they did (see Baker, 2003; 2005). Often students are also asked to self-monitor whether or not they enacted the skill steps, as self-monitoring may lead to better generalization. In addition to training parents and teachers to prompt students, peer training has also been used as a method to help generalize skills to natural settings.

Peer Sensitivity Training

When students with ASD have little opportunity to interact with peers, or worse yet, they are being teased, it is critical that training of "typical" peers become part of the social skills intervention. Peers can be taught to be "helpers" or coaches to students with autism during play or work times (see Dunn, 2005). They can also be taught to be good "bystanders," taking a protective role when their disabled peers are teased or bullied (see Baker, 2003; 2005). In addition, they can participate in social skills groups with their peers with autism to provide opportunities to interact in conversation and play.

For students with little symbolic language, I almost always involve typical peers. It can be quite challenging to get two children with limited attention and language to attend and interact with each other, but much easier to teach typical peers ways to engage those students. In addition, typical peers may be more flexible in their willingness to engage in our targeted student's preferred activities. One of the challenges for many children with autism is that their schools may not have access to typically developing peers. In these cases, it may be important to try to create relationships with nearby schools or community centers such as places of worship for access to typical peers.

Peer sensitivity training often begins with instructing peers on the strengths and challenges of students with social needs, and may include teaching about the symptoms of autism, or sometimes just about the needs of students who might be shy or need help socializing. After this training workshop, peers are solicited to become volunteer participants in socialization groups, lunchtime groups, or helpers at recess or during class and homework times. Descriptions of such programs can be found in my social skill manuals (Baker, 2003; Baker, 2005), as well as in other resources (Wagner, 1998; Dunn, 2005; Hughs & Carter, 2008).

Case Examples

Youngster with Symbolic Language Difficulties

Doug was a 6-year-old boy with classic autism. He attended a self-contained first grade class in a public school. He had limited functional language, including the ability to request certain foods and favored items, but could not yet converse about the past or future. His parents and teachers prioritized several skill goals based on their observations of what he did too much of and too little of. What he did too much of was demonstrating noncompliance and self-injurious behaviors (biting and hitting himself) when confronted with academic tasks. What he did too little of was initiating, responding to others' initiations, or sustaining playful interactions with peers.

Target Goals: 1) To ask for help rather than refuse academic tasks or hurt himself. 2) To initiate and respond to peers' initiations to play. 3) To sustain play for 10- to 20-minute periods of time with peers.

Motivational Issues: To increase Doug's motivation to do schoolwork, tasks were modified to ensure easier tasks were presented prior to challenging ones. In addition, the child's interest in animals was incorporated into academic materials in order to increase his interest in the tasks (e.g., math concepts were taught by counting toy animals).

To address motivation to initiate, respond to other's initiations, and sustain play, a variety of activities were introduced to explore what Doug would be intrinsically motivated to play. Because he likes animals, we began with an imitation game in which we modeled being an animal and then prompted him to imitate being that animal. For example, we walked on all fours and meowed or barked. Then we turned that into a "guess the animal" game in which we took turns guessing the animal someone was acting out. Doug smiled and seemed to enjoy playing these games. We also introduced other interactive games, such as hide and seek, red light/green light, and musical chairs. As Doug initially was not motivated to try these activities, we used the animal guessing game as an extrinsic reward, writing on a dry erase board, "first hide and seek, then play animals." As we tried these new games, he showed interest in hide and seek and red light/green light, but not musical chairs. Now we had established motivation for three games: guess the animal, hide and seek, and red light/green light.

Skill Acquisition: To teach Doug how to initiate and respond to play, we showed him the list of games he liked using pictures and words, and then asked him, "Do you want to play _____?" We prompted him to say, "I want to play _____" using whatever game he pointed to. We then continued to play until he became distracted, at which time we reintroduced the list of games and prompted, "Do you want to play _____ or take a break?" listing all the games and a picture of his break area.

To teach Doug how to ask for help instead of refusing to do work, we showed him a picture icon of what to do when work is hard. The picture showed a sample of work, and then two choices: 1) a happy face was depicted next to "ask for help" (a picture of a boy asking for help) or 2) a sad face next to a boy hitting himself. Then Doug was given work and whenever he became frustrated, he was directed to the visual icon and prompted to ask for help. Immediately, the teacher would either simplify the work or model how to do it. Video was also taken of Doug in which he was depicted asking for help with work. This video was then used as a primer before difficult work.

Generalization: To generalize play skills, we had typical peers come join Doug in play (two at a time, so they always had a friend with them for support). We instructed the peers to show Doug the visual list of games and ask him, "What do you want to play?" We also prompted Doug to say, "I want to play _____." His interaction with peers also provided opportunities for him to practice greetings and goodbyes. We provided these phrases and lists of games to his parents and his aide so that he could practice the skills and games at recess and at home with siblings or invited guests. His parents and aide were asked to come observe our sessions with peers so that they could replicate the prompting of skills on their own.

To generalize asking for help, parents and teachers were trained to re-direct Doug to ask for help using the visual card created. They also played the video of Doug asking for help prior to beginning each school day or doing difficult tasks at home.

Peer Sensitivity: With Doug's parents' permission, we conducted a peer sensitivity lesson in the regular first grade class with the students with whom Doug interacted at lunch and recess. They learned about Doug's strengths (e.g., interests in animals) as well as the strengths of a variety of famous people with autism. They also learned about the challenges of having autism, such as difficulty communicating and playing with others. They were asked to be peer buddies, coming into Doug's class twice per week with a friend to help him learn to play, and to engage him at recess. They were taught how to gain Doug's attention by asking him to look at them, and then they learned what kind of games Doug likes to play.

Outcome: Behavioral observations of play times indicated that Doug increased unprompted responses to peers and initiations to peers, and was able to sustain play for 15-minute periods. In terms of academic frustrations, overall Doug increased his requests for help and the frequency of hitting himself decreased. However, his responses varied depending on the level of difficulty or work presented to him.

Youngster with Excellent Symbolic Language

Peter was a 6th grader with Asperger syndrome. His academic skills were excellent, yet he had difficulty making friends and was often isolated from his peers, particularly at lunch and recess. He often did not edit himself and would say insulting things to others without realizing the impact it might have on them. In addition, he tended to talk obsessively about his interest in certain video games regardless of whether his listeners were interested.

Target Goals: Peter's parents and teachers prioritized several skill goals based on their observations of what he did too much of and too little of. What they agreed he did too much of was saying everything that was on his mind, including insulting remarks, and perseverating on his own interests. What they felt he did not do enough of was listening to others or asking about others. We articulated the following goals: 1) Avoid sensitive topics (i.e., insults, information not meant for public expression—such as violent talk from video games); 2) Initiate conversation based on common interests or interests relevant to peers; 3) Maintain conversation by asking or telling about what others just said; and 4) Check to see if others want to hear more if talking about favored interests (video games).

Motivational Issues: Peter was aware that he had few friends and expressed interest in having friends with whom to hang out. Looking at the motivational strategies in Table 2, we chose to focus on some of the intrinsic strategies for students with excellent symbolic language. We explained to Peter the rationale for learning to edit sensitive remarks and converse about common interests rather than perseverate on his own interests—i.e., that it would lead to greater opportunities for friendship. However, as for many students, we knew that a discussion of his skill challenges might feel like a criticism. Thus, we decided to first focus on his talents and strengths in academics and the strong future he will have, given these abilities. Then we explained that there were certain minor social issues to work on so that these talents could shine.

For the most part, Peter expressed motivation to focus on common interests with others and check to see if listeners wanted to talk about his favored video games. However, he was not always keen on editing sensitive remarks, as he often thought these comments were funny despite efforts to explain the negative impact his insults had on others. Thus, we added some extrinsic motivation strategies, making access to video games at home contingent on refraining from insulting others in school, as reported on a behavior chart that was sent home each night.

Skill Acquisition: The primary strategy to teach all skills was structured learning, in which we: 1) explained the rationale for learning the skill (the positive impact on making friends, or negative impact of not using the skills), 2) modeled the skill steps, 3) role-played the steps, and then 4) planned for transfer training (see the next section on generalization). Loose scripts for starting and maintaining conversation were pulled from my social skills manual (Baker, 2003). We taught these skills individually and then in a "lunch bunch" group with typical peers so that Peter had opportunities to practice these skills with peers.

Generalization: A weekly lunch bunch group with typical peers allowed Peter to be coached on good conversation skill while conversing with typical peers. In addition, cue cards containing these loose scripts were provided to his teachers and parents with instructions as to how to prime these skills prior to social opportunities. Peter did not want his parents or teachers observing lunch bunch, so we had individual conferences with parents and teachers so they could learn how to prime and coach these skills.

According to the research, 30 hours of this kind of group training over 12 weeks may not be enough to create change, yet the reality of the school's staff availability left us with a once-a-week group that lasted 40 minutes. However, lunch bunch members were encouraged to eat with each other on non-lunch bunch days as well. Each day Peter's teacher primed the conversation skills prior to lunch and Peter filled out a brief self-monitoring sheet after lunch to indicate whether he had initiated conversation based on common interests and refrained from any insulting remarks. In addition, in every class, Peter was rated on his ability to refrain from uttering insensitive remarks to others, and the information was recorded on a behavior chart. That chart went home each day and determined how much video game time he could have each night.

Peer Sensitivity: Peter did not want his peers to know he had an autism spectrum disorder. So in soliciting volunteers for a lunch bunch group, we did not talk about Peter specifically to his peers. Instead we spoke to the entire 6th grade class about all students feeling lonely at times if they are new to the school, are shy, or need some help socializing. We offered the opportunity for all the 6th graders to attend a weekly lunch bunch group on a rotating basis so that anyone who wanted to could attend the group. Peter attended each time. If anyone questioned why he was there each time, we indicated that his parents wanted him to have the opportunity to eat in a quieter area once a week rather than in the loud cafeteria.

Outcome: Based on baseline ratings from parents and teachers, Peter "rarely" avoided sensitive topics, initiated conversation on common interests, or maintained conversation with follow-up questions. At the end of 16 weeks, average ratings of these skills were rated as "often" to "almost always," indicating improvement from his parents' and teachers' perspectives. These changes did not automatically result in more friendships for Peter. Yet by contacting some of the peers' parents, we were able to set up some after school play dates, which resulted in more regular get-togethers with students who then considered Peter to be a friend.

References

Baker, J. E. (2008). *No more meltdowns.* Arlington, TX: Future Horizons.

Baker, J .E. (2007*). Social skills training and frustration management.* [DVD]. Arlington, TX: Future Horizons. Order through www.fhautism.com.

Baker, J .E. (2006). *The social skills picture book for high school and beyond.* Arlington, TX: Future Horizons.

Baker, J. E. (2005). *Preparing for life: The complete guide to transitioning to adulthood for those with autism and Aspergers syndrome.* Arlington, TX: Future Horizons.

Baker, J. E. (2003). *Social skills training for students with Aspergers syndrome and related social communication disorders.* Shawnee Mission, Kansas: Autism Aspergers Publishing Company.

Baker, J. E. (2001). *Social skills picture books.* Arlington, TX: Future Horizons.

Bellini, S., & Akullian, J. (2007). A meta-analysis of video modeling and video self-modeling interventions for children and adolescents with autism spectrum disorders. *Exceptional Children, 73,* 261-284.

Bellini, S., Akullian, J., & Hopf, A. (2007). Increasing social engagement in young children with autism spectrum disorders using video self-modeling. *School Psychology Review, 36,* 80-90.

Bellini, S., Peters, J., Benner, L., & Hopf, A. (2007). A meta-analysis of school-based social skills interventions for children with autism spectrum disorders. *Remedial and Special Education, 28*(3), 153-162.

Bellini, S., & Peters, J. (2008). Social skills training for youth with autism spectrum disorders. *Child and Adolescent Psychiatric Clinics of North America, 17,* 857-873.

Dawson, G., Rogers, S., Munson, J., Smith, M., Winter, J., Greenson, J., Donaldson, A., & Varley, J. (2009, Nov. 30). Randomized, controlled trial of an intervention for toddlers with autism: The Early Start Denver Model. *Pediatrics.* [Epub ahead of print]. PubMed PMID: 19948568.

Dunn, M. (2005*). S.O.S. Social skills in our schools: A social skill program for children with pervasive developmental disorders, including high-functioning autism and Asperger syndrome, and their typical peers.* Shawnee Mission, Kansas: Autism Aspergers Publishing Company.

Frost, L., & Bondy, A. (2006). A common language: Using B.F. Skinner's verbal behavior for assessment and treatment of communication disabilities in SLP-ABA. *The Journal of Speech-Language Pathology and Applied Behavior Analysis, 1,* 103-110.

Greenspan, S., & Wieder, S. (1998). *The child with special needs: Encouraging intellectual and emotional growth.* Reading, MA: Addison Wesley Longman.

Greenspan, S.I., & Wieder, S. (2005). Can children with autism master the core deficits and become empathetic, creative and reflective? A ten to fifteen year follow-up of a subgroup of children with autism spectrum disorders (ASD) who received a comprehensive developmental, individual-difference, relationship-based (DIR) approach. *The Journal of Developmental and Learning Disorders, 9.*

Gresham, F. M., Sugai, G., & Horner, R. H. (2001). Interpreting outcomes of social skills training for students with high-incidence disabilities. *Exceptional Children, 67*, 331-344.

Gutstein, S. E., & Sheely, R. K. (2002). *Relationship development intervention with children, adolescents, and adults: Social and emotional development activities for Asperger syndrome, autism, PDD, and NLD.* London: Jessica Kingsley Publishers.

Gutstein, S. E. (2007). Evaluation of the Relationship Development Intervention Program. *Autism, 11*(5), 397–411.

Harlow, H. F. (1962). Development of affection in primates. In E.L. Bliss (Ed.), *Roots of Behavior.* New York, NY: Harper.

Hughes, C., & Carter, E. W. (2008). *Peer buddy programs for successful secondary school inclusion.* Baltimore, MD: Paul H. Brookes.

Kaufman, B. N. (1994). *Son-Rise: The miracle Vontinues.* Tiburon, CA: H. J. Kramer.

Koegel, R. L., & Koegel, L. K. (2006). *Pivotal response treatments for autism: Communication, social, & academic development.* Baltimore, MD: Paul H. Brookes.

Lovaas, O. I. (1987). Behavioral treatment and normal educational and intellectual functioning in young autistic children. *Journal of Consulting & Clinical Psychology, 55*, 3-9.

Mesibov, G. B., Shea, V., & Schopler, E. (with Adams, L., Burgess, S., Chapman, S. M., Merkler, E., Mosconi, M., Tanner, C., & Van Bourgondien, M. E.). (2005). *The TEACCH approach to autism spectrum disorders.* New York: Kluwer Academic/Plenum.

Sundberg, M. L., & Partington, J. W. (1998). *Teaching language to children with autism or other developmental disabilities.* Pleasant Hill, CA: Behavior Analysts.

Trimarchi, C. L. (2004). The implementation and evaluation of a social skills training program for children with Asperger syndrome. Unpublished doctoral dissertation, University at Albany, State University of New York.

Wagner, S. (1998). *Inclusive programming for elementary students with autism.* Arlington, TX: Future Horizons.

White, S. W., Koenig, K., & Scahill, L.(2006). Social skills development in children with autism spectrum disorders: A review of the intervention research. *Journal of Autism and Developmental Disorders, 37*(10). http://dx.doi.org/ 10.1007/s10803-006-0320-x.

Winner, M. G. (2004). *Think social! A social thinking curriculum for school-age students.* San Jose, CA: Think Social Publishing.

8

Social Skills:
Strategies and Challenges
Mary Jane Weiss

Social skills are agreed upon as centrally important in instructing individuals on the autism spectrum. They are, however, among the most elusive targets to impact. One challenge to teaching such skills is that learners with autism spectrum disorders (ASD) may have minimal intrinsic interest in learning these skills. Many learners with ASD lack social interest, have constricted social interests, have difficulties following social rules, and/or fail to comprehend social nuances. Additionally, they often exhibit little social initiation, as well as reduced social responsiveness. In summary, it is not difficult to understand the instructional challenges when we examine the diagnostic features and the motivational issues. One of the reasons clinicians struggle in this context is that social skills are *particularly* and *uniquely* challenging to individuals with autism.

Furthermore, it is often difficult to conceptualize how to instruct individuals with autism in such skills. Most social skills are multi-element skills that require the individual to engage in several different and distinct tasks. Consider turn taking. We could list many different discrete skills required for successful turn taking. These include: listening to directions, inhibiting actions, following rules, understanding cues for action and non-action, delay of gratification, etc.

Perhaps most importantly, most of the skills in the social realm involve an element of judgment (i.e., is it appropriate to engage in this behavior with this person at this time?). These varying situational elements and instructional complexities make it difficult to teach such skills. How does one define social judgment so it can be measured and is it even possible to do so? Furthermore, how can we program for generalization of these skills? Is it even possible to prepare learners for the myriad possibilities that exist in real life?

This chapter will review these challenges to definition and to instruction, some of the ways in which such skills are commonly taught to individuals on the autism spectrum, and some broad issues that relate to the utility of these skills.

We have already reviewed some of the issues in definition. The core issues revolve around defining social skills in a functional context. What is a social skill? Is it simply a skill that is expected in society? Is it a skill that increases navigation independently? Is it a skill that prevents negative consequences? In other words, are social skills really rules about what *not* to do?

The chapters in this book present several frameworks for defining and teaching social skills. While there are differences in authors' views, each chapter presents a pragmatic approach to enhancing social functioning.

Instructional Challenges

There are several ways that social skills are approached in instructional contexts. Often, a skill will be discussed as a curricular area, as in play skills. Such an area may be broken down into stages and sub-stages of instructions, with corollary and corresponding programs. At times, a core or pivotal skill may be focused on as a distinct skill or progression of skills. For example, Theory of Mind or perspective taking is often discussed in this way. These elegant interventions provide an operationally defined set of procedures and a clear instructional progression.

In practice, however, social skills are often targeted in a multipronged approach. Many commonly used approaches are packaged interventions with several components that are used in combination with other procedures. Weiss and Harris (2001) provide a thorough description of several strategies for teaching social skills to young children on the autism spectrum.

Unfortunately, many commonly used strategies have limited empirical support to date. Additionally, some approaches have been empirically supported with different populations, but not with individuals on the autism spectrum. (For example, systematic problem-solving curricula have been successful in teaching problem-solving skills to children with ADHD.) The utility of these interventions is unclear, but many clinicians use procedures from other populations to address higher-level social skills. Several commercially available social skills chapters and curricula have well-formulated and clear lessons for a variety of social skill instructional targets (e.g., Baker, 2002; 2003; McGinnis & Goldstein, 1990; Richardson, 1996; Taylor, 2001; Taylor & Jasper, 2001).

In clinical application, a number of commonly used strategies fit the descriptions above (i.e., they have limited empirical support or have been used primarily with other types of learners). Nevertheless, such procedures are often used to remediate social deficits and to teach social skills. Importantly, they are often used in combination with other, direct behavior change procedures, such as reinforcement and prompting. Examples of such commonly used procedures that will be reviewed here include Social Stories, role-plays, rule cards, scripts, and video modeling. This review is designed to provide examples of the challenges that exist both in our empirical literature and in our guidelines for clinical practice. The procedures described are commonly used as parts of multi-component or package approaches to behavior reduction and skill acquisition. As such, it can be difficult to isolate the effects of any one component. This is a major problem in the empirical verification of procedures used in social skills instruction.

Commonly Used Techniques
Social Stories

Social Stories™ are an intervention developed by Carol Gray (Gray, 1993; 1994) that provide information about social situations and about behavior that is expected in those situations. Gray has suggested a formula or ratio of one directive statement to every three to five informational statements. This ratio is designed to ensure that the story convey information about complex or hard-to-comprehend social circumstances.

Social Stories can be written in various ways. Many clinicians combine text with pictures, and some clinicians make the stories extremely individualized (including using the names of people the individual knows and using the first person). The stories are used to convey information and expectations for multi-element tasks (such as cleaning up or lining up for recess). They are often used as part of a group of interventions to reduce challenging behaviors, and offer functional alternatives to the target behavior, such as asking for help instead of throwing materials.

There is some encouraging empirical support for the effectiveness of Social Stories in increasing social communication skills (e.g., Thiemann & Goldstein, 2001). However, the data are quite variable and knowledge is limited (Reynhout & Carter, 2006). Some of the problems that exist in the current body of literature include: highly variable effect sizes, highly variable methodology, and a lack of reports of cognitive level of individuals in the studies.

Even in a clinical context, there are more questions than answers. Many clinical aspects of the use of Social Stories remain unanswered from a research perspective. It does not appear that there is an effect for descriptive sentences (Reynout and Carter, 2006). Little is known about most other elements of story construction or clinical implementation. It is not known how frequently reviews of the story need to be done, whether comprehension activities make it easier for learners to master the content, or the best schedule for presentation of the story. The data are not robust with regard to the ability of Social Stories to facilitate behavioral change. Furthermore, data on the maintenance and generalization of such changes are largely unavailable. Given that maintenance and generalization are critical issues for individuals with ASD, this is a serious limitation.

However, consumers like Social Stories, are enthusiastic about including them in curricular planning, and are fairly compliant about implementing them. There are also many anecdotal reports of success with their use. The question for the clinician is whether, how, and when to use them. It may be possible and advantageous to use them as part of a package/group of interventions, as long as more direct change procedures are also used. However, the responsible behavior analyst would want to know whether, how, and how much Social Stories are contributing to behavior change in the individuals with whom they are working.

Role Plays

Role plays provide an opportunity for the rehearsal of desired behaviors (e. g., Snell & Janney, 2000; Weiss & Harris, 2001). We know that students with ASD often need multiple opportunities to learn and to practice desired skills. Hence, role plays may naturally provide such additional opportunities and supplement a low number of naturally occurring events in the natural environment.

Role plays can be used to target elements and nuances of interaction that are central to social success. Examples include orientating to the speaker, maintaining eye contact, and answering questions appropriately. Role plays can be done in different ways, with characters, puppets, people, and the target student. When the student participates, he or she can take on different roles, demonstrating the initial skill or the response. Role plays are always used together with feedback on performance. While there is not a body of research on role-play procedures, there is some support for the broad use of behavioral rehearsal strategies. This is one of the strategies that has been demonstrated to be effective with populations other than individuals with autism, and may be relevant.

Rule Cards

Rule cards assist students in following the social rules that are associated with a particular activity (e.g., Weiss & Harris, 2001). A rule card states the specific behavioral expectations for an activity. Rule cards are sometimes reviewed prior to an activity and can also be used in combination with other procedures (such as behavioral rehearsal). Rule cards are very helpful for targeting skills such as taking turns, sharing materials, and asking peers for items. They can also be used for delineating behavioral expectations for a particular environment or activity, such as the library or school assemblies. While there is not a body of literature on the use of rule cards *per se,* they are a common clinical intervention and are related to a variety of visual prompting strategies and behavioral rehearsal techniques that have been shown to be effective (e.g., Cooper, Heron, & Heward, 2007; Snell & Brown, 2000).

Scripts

Many students with autism have a difficult time engaging in conversations, even if they have well-developed language comprehension. They may also have difficulty in creative play. In both conversations and creative play, it is difficult to predict what other individuals will do, so the demands for flexibility are high. As a result of their deficits, individuals with autism may engage in much less interaction than they might appear to be capable of. One way to address this issue is to provide scripts for conversations or creative play. Scripts can be provided in the form of sentences, words, or pictures, and they can be used in a variety of circumstances (e.g., Snell & Janney, 2000). Scripts can also be specifically developed for a particular context, game, or activity. Scripts can help the learner to engage in the target behavior for longer durations. Also, they can assist the learner in staying on topic and engaged while involved in interaction. A number of studies document the effectiveness of scripts, including in facilitating social initiation and social interaction (e.g., Krantz & McClannahan, 1993, 1998).

Rote behavior or rigidity can be a concern whenever scripts are used. It is therefore important to program in variability in the script and to reinforce flexibility in the response. It is not functional if the learner can speak about a topic in only one way or play with a toy in only one unchanging sequence. We need to prepare individuals with ASD for the wide variety of circumstances they are likely to encounter in their interactions, and we need to build their capacity and tolerance for change.

Video Modeling

Video modeling, which is described in the chapter by Rebecca MacDonald, is an area where more research literature does exist. Video modeling has been shown to be a very effective means of teaching students with ASD to imitate peers (Haring, Kennedy, Adams, & Pitts-Conway, 1987), learn sign language (Watkins, Sprafkin, & Krolikowski, 1993), develop play skills (Charlop-Christy, Le, & Freeman, 2000), and develop conversation skills (Charlop & Milstein, 1989; Sherer et al., 2001). Increasingly, video modeling is being used successfully to build a variety of skills, including functional academic skills, community-relevant skills, conversational exchanges, and play skills (e.g., Snell & Brown, 2000; Taylor, 2001; Weiss & Harris, 2001). The literature about its effectiveness is compelling and robust.

The use of video is also clinically appealing, as many students with ASD are strong visual learners and enjoy watching videos. There has been speculation that individuals with autism may attend better to a model presented in a video clip than they would to a live model demonstrating a skill. Clinically, video modeling is often presented as an adult demonstrating the skill first. When using an adult model, it may be easier to ensure that the important aspects of the target behavior are made salient. In addition, older peers or mature peers can be used as models. These individuals have inherent advantages, because of their similarities to the target students.

Video modeling has been used to teach a variety of play skills. While there is some variability in how video modeling is implemented to build play skills, it usually involves having learners observe a clip and then enact the demonstrated skills themselves. There may be a phase of concurrent imitation of the behavior (doing the actions along with the model on tape), followed by a phase of delayed imitation of the observed behavior (watching the clip and then playing). The rote nature of the response is a concern, so it is important to program in variability. The learner can also be eventually rewarded for expanding upon or varying the modeled skills.

In addition, the video medium can be used to provide feedback to learners on their performance. Both reinforcement and corrective feedback can be provided, and the experience can be used to develop better skills. Specifically, strategies for targeted areas of weakness can be modeled and rehearsed (e.g., Taylor, 2001). This may be an especially useful strategy for situations in which an individual has demonstrated difficulty understanding social rules, such as respecting personal space or staying on topic in a conversation.

Guidelines for the use of video with students with ASD have been developed (e.g., Krantz, MacDuff, Wadstrom, & McClannahan, 1991). Specifically, these authors suggest: assessing learners for necessary prerequisite skills; removing extraneous stimuli from the environment; factoring in the history of the learner with the people who are presenting the video or modeling on the video; and considering cognitive level as a possible prerequisite (as learners with more developed cognitive skills may have better outcomes). You may also wish to refer to *Seeing Is Believing: Video Self-Modeling for People with Autism and Other Developmental Disabilities* by Tom Buggey (Woodbine House, 2009).

Problem Solving

The capacity to solve problems is an important part of success in school, at work, in interpersonal relationships, and in life. Problem solving is also critically important to the social world of friendships. Many students with social skills difficulties due to other types of problems, such as ADHD, have benefited substantially from problem-solving approaches.

Problem-solving training generally includes helping learners to both identify problems and select appropriate solutions. Children with ASD often have difficulties with identifying the social problem. This may be due to the apparent ambiguity of presenting problems. They also struggle with evaluating options for a course of action. They may be impulsive and quickly act on the first option that comes to mind, or they may simply fail to see the range of options. Training in problem-solving (e.g., Shure, 2001a; 2001b; 2004) can help students with ASD to identify problems, generate alternative solutions, evaluate the effectiveness of different possible paths of action, and choose the best option (Bieber, 1994; Dunn, 2006). This approach is flexible, and can be done as a class-wide intervention or as an individual approach.

Evaluating Social Significance

As behavior analysts, we always discuss the importance of socially significant change. Nowhere in curricular programming is this more important than in the realm of social skills. Issues of social significance center on the meaningfulness of behavior change. It is not meaningful if the skill is demonstrated in an isolated context. It is also not meaningful if the skill is not demonstrated in a functional way. For example, if the duration or latency for a behavior is excessive, the learner will not receive reinforcement in a maximally effective way. Thus, a child with autism may miss out on the chance to interact with a friend if it takes him too long to respond to a greeting.

Generalization is an issue of central importance in social skills. There is little use in teaching conversation in a scripted way unless the learner eventually tolerates unscripted interactions. Similarly, with play skills, students need to respond to different fire stations, garages, farms, and dollhouses. Our attention to generality needs to permeate our social skills programming. We need to remember the lessons of Stokes and Baer (1977), who emphasized the use of multiple exemplars, the importance of training loosely, and the strategy of varying elements of the instructional context to facilitate the transfer of skills.

Similarly, we need to attend to time-based dimensions of behavior when teaching social skills. Duration and latency are salient features of social interactions. Deficits in the stamina and responsiveness of learners have severe social consequences. Consequently, building speed of response is critically important.

Summary of Clinical Approaches

It is difficult to specify what is meant by social skills. Many behavior analysts single out particular skills (e.g., joint attention or play) that can be targeted as a curricular progression. In these elegant progressions, one can see the basic tenets of ABA in action, including operational definitions, clear criteria for mastery, and a sequenced instructional approach.

In clinical practice, however, a variety of techniques are commonly used for teaching social skills to individuals with autism spectrum disorders. Many of the techniques that are commonly used are not empirically validated or have been used primarily with other populations. They may, however, be useful additional components to a package of behavioral interventions. They are often implemented in this way—as one element of a multi-element approach. Such packaged interventions may improve the learner's acquisition of these multi-element skills. At the least, they may provide more practice/learning opportunities and increase the extent to which individuals with ASD are prepared for the range of possible experiences.

In consideration of the use of non-verified treatments or packaged interventions, it is important that direct behavior-change procedures always be used to affect behavior. In addition, data on the effectiveness of all strategies used with individual learners should always be collected to make it easier to make data-based decisions about the continuation or discontinuation of any treatments or any components of treatments.

In all social skills programming, our emphasis must be on the mastery of behaviors that have true social significance. Toward that end, we must program for generality in the stimuli we select, the settings we instruct in, the teaching procedures we use, and the responses that we reinforce. We must also attend to the issue of response availability. Students with ASD must respond in a timely way to peer initiation, as failing to do so will result in fewer social bids.

In the curricular realm of social skills, functionality must be our barometer of effectiveness. Do the skills we teach make a real-world difference for this individual? Does he or she now have greater access to reinforcement? Does he have fewer negative interactions? Can he navigate social contexts more easily? Is the learner more independent? Has he found a community of individuals who share his interests? The focus is on ultimate outcomes. Our teaching strategies must reflect and be shaped by this goal.

References

Baker, J. E. (2003). *Social skills training.* Shawnee Mission, KS: Autism Asperger Publishing Co.

Baker, J. E. (2003). *Social skills picture book: Teaching play, emotion, and communication to children with autism.* Arlington, TX: Future Horizons.

Bieber, J. (1994). *Learning disabilities and social skills with Richard Lavoie: Last one picked . . . first one picked on.* Washington, DC: Public Broadcasting Service.

Charlop, M. H., & Milstein, J. P. (1989). Teaching autistic children conversational speech using video modeling. *Journal of Applied Behavior Analysis, 22,* 275-285.

Charlop-Christy, M. H., Le, L., & Freeman, K. A. (2000). A comparison of video modeling with in vivo modeling for teaching children with autism. *Journal of Autism and Developmental Disorders, 30,* 537-552.

Cooper, J. O., Heron, T. E., & Heward, W. L. (2007). *Applied behavior analysis* (2nd ed.). Upper Saddle River, NJ: Prentice Hall.

Dunn, M. (2006). *S. O. S.: Social Skills in Our Schools: A social skills program for children with pervasive developmental disorders, including high functioning autism and Asperger syndrome and their typical peers.* Shawnee Mission, KS: Autism Asperger Publishing Company.

Gray, C. (1993). *The original Social Story book.* Arlington, TX: Future Horizons.

Gray, C. (1994). *The new Social Story book.* Arlington, TX: Future Horizons.

Haring, T., Kennedy, C., Adams, M., & Pitts-Conway, V. (1987). Teaching generalization of purchasing skills across community settings to autistic youth using videotape modeling. *Journal of Applied Behavior Analysis, 20,* 89-96.

Krantz, P. J., MacDuff, G. S., Wadstrom, O., & McClannahan, L. E. (1991). Using video with developmentally disabled learners. In P. W. Dowrick (Ed.), *Practical guide to video in the behavioral sciences* (pp. 256-266). New York, NY: John Wiley & Sons.

Krantz, P. J., & McClannahan, L. E. (1993). Teaching children with autism to initiate to peers: Effects of a script-fading procedure. *Journal of Applied Behavior Analysis, 26,* 121-132.

Krantz , P. J., & McClannahan, L. E. (1998). Social interaction skills for children with autism: A script-fading procedure for beginning readers. *Journal of Applied Behavior Analysis, 31,* 191-202.

McGinnis, E., & Goldstein, A. P. (1990). *Skillstreaming.* Champaign, IL: Research Press.

Reynhout, G., & Carter, M. (2006). Social stories for children with disabilities. *Journal of Autism and Developmental Disorders, 36,* 445-469.

Richardson, R. C. (1996). *Connecting with others: Lessons for teaching social and emotional competence.* Champaign, IL: Research Press.

Sherer, M., Pierce, K. L., Parades, S., Kisacky, K. L., Ingersoll, B., & Schreibman, L. (2001). Enhancing conversation skills in children with autism via video technology: Which is better, "self" or "other" as a model. *Behavior Modification, 25,* 140-158.

Shure, M. B. (2001a). *I can problem solve (kindergarten and primary grades).* Champaign, IL: Research Press.

Shure, M. B. (2001b). *I can problem solve (intermediate elementary grades).* Champaign, IL: Research Press.

Shure, M. B. (2004). *I can problem solve (preschool).* Champaign, IL: Research Press.

Snell, M. E., & Brown, F. (2000). *Instruction of students with severe handicaps.* Upper Saddle River, NJ: Prentice Hall.

Snell, M. E., & Janney, R. (2000). *Social relationships and peer support.* Baltimore, MD: Paul H. Brookes.

Taylor, B. A. (2001). Teaching peer social skills to children with autism. In C. Maurice, G. Green, & R. Foxx (Eds.), *Making a difference: Behavioral intervention for autism* (pp. 83-96). Austin, TX: Pro-Ed.

Taylor, B. A., & Jasper, S. (2001). Teaching programs to increase peer interaction. In C. Maurice, G. Green, & R. Foxx (Eds.), *Making a Difference: Behavioral Intervention for Autism* (pp. 97-162). Austin, TX: Pro-Ed.

Thiemann, K. S., & Goldstein, H. (2001). Social stories, written text cues, and video feedback: Effects on social communication of children with autism. *Journal of Applied Behavior Analysis, 34,* 425-446.

Watkins, L. T., Sprafkin, J. N., & Krolikowski, D. M. (1993). Using videotaped lessons to facilitate the development of manual sign skills in students with mental retardation. *Augmentative and Alternative Communication, 9,* 177-183.

Weiss, M. J., & Harris, S. L. (2001). *Reaching out, joining in: Teaching social skills to young children with autism.* Bethesda, MD: Woodbine House.

Contributors

Shahla Ala'i-Rosales, Ph.D., BCBA-D
Associate Professor
Department of Behavior Analysis
University of North Texas
Denton, Texas

Jed Baker, Ph.D.
Director
The Social Skills Project
Locations in New York and New Jersey

Andy Bondy, Ph.D.
Cofounder and President
Pyramid Educational Consultants
Newark, Delaware

Samantha Marie Cermak, M.S., BCBA
The Homestead Autism Services
Altoona, Iowa

Marjorie Charlop, Ph.D.
Professor and Director of the Claremont Autism Center
Claremont McKenna College
Claremont, California

Melaura Andree Erickson, Ph.D., BCBA-D
Claremont Graduate University
Claremont, California

Kristín Guðmundsdóttir, M.S., BCBA
Assistant Professor
Department of Social Sciences
School of Humanities and Social Sciences
University of Akureyri, Iceland

Connie Kasari, Ph.D.
Professor
University of California at Los Angeles
Los Angeles, California

Saara Mahjouri, Ph.D.
Postdoctoral Fellow in Psychology
Weill Cornell Medical College
White Plains, NY

Rebecca MacDonald, Ph.D., BCBA-D
Program Director
New England Center for Children
Southborough, Massachusetts and London

Daniel Openden, Ph.D., BCBA-D
President and CEO
Southwest Autism Research and Resource Center
Phoenix, Arizona

Bridget A. Taylor, PsyD, BCBA-D
Cofounder and Executive Director
Alpine Learning Group
Paramus, New Jersey

Mary Jane Weiss, Ph.D., BCBA-D
Professor and Director of Programs in ABA and Autism
Endicott College
Beverly, Massachusetts

Index

About the Editors:

Andy Bondy is a behavior analyst and co-developer of PECS. He co-founded Pyramid Education Consultants, Inc., an internationally based team promoting functional communication and functional skills for everyone.

Many Jane Weiss is Professor of Education and the director of Programs in Autism and ABA at Endicott College. She conducts research at Melmark, an organization for people with disabilities.

4751012